Flatter Your Figure™

Flatter Your Figure™

JAN LARKEY

A FIRESIDE BOOK
Published by Simon & Schuster
New York London Toronto Sydney Tokyo Singapore

*This book is dedicated to every woman
who has a figure problem.*

FIRESIDE

Rockefeller Center
1230 Avenue of the Americas
New York, New York 10020

FIRESIDE and colophon are registered trademarks
of Simon & Schuster Inc.

Flatter Your Figure™ is a trademark of Jan Larkey
Designed by Nina D'Amario/Levavi & Levavi

Manufactured in the United States of America

15 16 17 18 19 20

First Fireside Edition 1992

Library of Congress Cataloging-in-Publication Data
Larkey, Jan.
Flatter your figure / Jan Larkey.—1st Prentice Hall ed.
p.   cm.
1. Clothing and dress.   2. Fashion.   3. Beauty, Personal.
I. Title.
TT507.L28   1991
646'.34—dc20   90-41155
ISBN: 0-671-76296-6   CIP

A Special Thanks

IN 1985, I ILLUSTRATED A FEW PAGES OF CLOTHING STYLES TO help some clients who were frustrated about finding clothes that flattered their figures. Colleagues started requesting a few copies. They all requested more information. By 1986 the idea of turning those few pages into a book that could help hundreds of women became my dream. The following people deserve special recognition for helping this dream come true.

To author Clare Revelli, whose success story dared me to think "BOOK"; to Angie Michaels and Chris and Sandy Smith who encouraged me to actually do it; to Carole Jackson and Leah Feldon for their insights into becoming an author; to Lenore Benson of The Fashion Group, Inc., and the Fashion Institute of Technology for research assistance.

To my special friends and professional colleagues: Susan Demme, Sally Horner, Mina Bancroft, Janet Lubic, Barbara Bogart, Mary Shellum, and Karla Jordan for inspiration and ideas; to the hundreds of professionals who used the earlier workbook and suggested how to improve it.

To those whose roles in the publishing process have made this book a joyful adventure: my editor Toni Sciarra, Editor-in-Chief Marilyn Abraham, and my agent Pam Bernstein.

To my family: Hank, Jana, Stephanie, and Carrie and to my mother, Dixie, for love and support . . . and to the man behind this woman, my incredible Patrick.

To Mary Sue Kamen and Janice Dolnack, my assistants, for extra help, time and time again.

To Cathy Guisewite the creator of "Cathy," the comic strip character whose "dressing room despair" helps us laugh at our figure and shopping problems.

And especially to all my wonderful clients with all those figure problems who started me on the quest to find the answers you will find on these pages . . .

To each of you, a fond, heartfelt *THANKS*.

I'm often asked how long it took to write and illustrate this book. My answer is "twenty years and nine months." The following people each contributed to my growth as an artist, educator, and consultant during those twenty years. Special appreciation goes to the Dutch artist Cor Vissor who taught me how to draw; the art professors at Texas Tech who taught me about design elements; Elliot Eisner at Stanford who taught me about sequential learning; and the founders of Color 1, JoAnne Nicholson and Judy Lewis Crum, who influenced my career change from art teacher to image consultant. The information on the use of color and accessories on pages 70, and 76–86 is based, in part, on the concepts they share in *Color Wonderful* (Bantam Books, 1986).

Contents

How Flatter Your Figure Is Designed to Help You

Have you ever seen a model or a mannequin with a shape like yours?

If your answer is NO, this book is for you.

If your answer is YES, this book is for you, too.

Why? Because even the most fabulous figure may appear to have problems when it is clothed in unflattering styles.

You are about to discover the secrets of how to put your figure and clothes together in the most flattering way possible. You will never again have to play the guessing game of wondering how a garment displayed on a model, mannequin, or in a catalog will look on *you*. So, get a pencil and get ready to:

FIGURE OUT YOUR FIGURE

Hide the measuring tape! A fascinating way to figure out your figure without measurements is revealed for the first time on pages 17–27. Step-by-step illustrations will show you and your friends exactly how to evaluate your figure using only two sticks and a string. Anyone can do it. It's fun. It's easy. Within minutes you will be able to see your figure as objectively as other people do.

FIGURE OUT FASHIONS

Do you ever wonder why some clothes make you look great, while others make you feel like you just gained 10 pounds? The answers are in Chapter 3.

Just follow the guidelines throughout this book to discover which styles are flattering, acceptable, or detracting for your own unique combination of figure challenges.

FLATTER YOUR FIGURE

You can see yourself as others see you—with just a blink of the eyes. Learning how to pass the Blink Test on pages 89–90 will have you feeling confident that all of the parts—you, your clothing, and your accessories—add up to a terrific look from head to toe.

Would you like to look taller? Thinner? The tendency to focus on inches, pounds, and sizes will be forgotten when you know how to create illusions with your clothing. Check out the "special strategies" section. Chapter 4 will show you how to make clothing combinations work—and even how to turn mistakes into flattering fashion statements.

ACCENT YOUR ASSETS

Learning how to camouflage figure problems is only the first step toward looking your best. Identifying your most positive features and learning how to create focal points that accent your assets will complete your figure analysis.

SHOP SUCCESSFULLY WITH YOUR FIGURE CHART

Flatter Your Figure (FYF) was written in a workbook format so that you can customize the information for your own figure. In the back of the book you will find a Figure Chart. It will become your own personalized guide to help you easily remember how too:

1. Camouflage figure problems
2. Buy, order, or sew your most flattering styles
3. Accent your assets—always

How long will it take to complete *FYF* for *your* figure?
Only about an hour.

How long can you use it?
All of your life.

Wishes, Magic, and Reality

CINDERELLA: A MAGICAL MAKE-OVER

Wouldn't shopping be wonderful if, instead of trudging from dressing room to dressing room, you could just ask Cinderella's fairy godmother to wave her magic wand, and—"P-o-o-oof"—you'd have a gorgeous body and wardrobe . . . all for the price of a pumpkin?

If you are like the thousands of women I have had the pleasure of working with as an image consultant since 1980, the chances are that your shopping frustrations start when you look in the mirror and wish that you could change your figure.

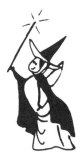

Easier wished than done.
Your wish may be to change your weight, have longer legs, thinner

thighs, to look like a model, or to look as good as you did five years ago.

In reality, the body you may wish you could magically change is often a challenge to dress in styles that truly flatter you. Like many of my clients, you may have a closet full of "guilt garments"—unworn mistakes representing wasted time and money.

Fret no more. In less time than it took you to purchase your last shopping mistake, you can complete this workbook and have a guide that will help you:

- Shop faster
- Save money
- Eliminate shopping, sewing, and mail-order mistakes
- Salvage mistakes already in your closet
- Get dressed each day knowing exactly what to add or change to look your best, and, last but not least,
- Look in your mirror and smile

MIRROR, MIRROR, ON THE WALL

I was eleven when I first looked in the mirror and really frowned.

As I stood looking in a full-length mirror in my new bathing suit, I noticed that I looked lopsided. "Look Mom, I'm crooked," I said. She glanced at me and dismissed my concerns with the suggestion, "Stand up straighter."

As the summer months went by, it soon became evident that my figure was starting to show some curves . . . but not in the usual places. I definitely *was* crooked! Within a short time, my body became so deformed that people stared, children pointed, and my exercise instructor used me as an example of how bad posture could lead to a deformed body. *Deformed*. The word echoed in my head and was confirmed in my mirror.

The doctors explained that a strange illness two years earlier had probably been a mild case of polio. The weakened muscles on one side of my spine had given way in the direction of the stronger muscles on the other side. The result: a major curvature of the spine. Rather than looking like a hunchback, I looked lopsided.

That is when I discovered that clothing could be my friend or foe. In some outfits I looked straighter; in others my deformity was more obvious. Straight skirts, for example, accented my lopsidedness because the hemline went up at a distinct angle. Little did I know then that the process of discovering how clothing can create illusions would become my area of expertise as an adult.

Fortunately, most of my curvature was straightened by surgically fusing six vertebrae. The procedure required that I be encased for nine months in a body cast: a plaster cocoon. I remember thinking, "Soon I'll have a straight back, then I'll look great. No one will tease me or call me deformed again!"

Do you sometimes think, "If only I could change_____, then I would like my body?"

The day finally came for me to emerge from the cast. As the plaster was cut away, I looked down at my straight body. Straight was certainly the word to describe me. There wasn't a curve in sight! Straightening my back had added four inches to my height. I was now 5 feet, 7 inches tall but weighed only 104 pounds. I looked anorexic.

I was thrilled about not being deformed anymore, but I was still upset about my figure. In the year I had been getting straightened out, all my friends had been developing curves . . . in the right places! I looked at their figures, especially Sue's. (Remember that lucky girl with the gorgeous body from your teen years?) Compared to Sue, I looked like Twiggy, a top model of the 1960s, whose skinny shape would be in vogue several years in the future. (The then-current movie idol was curvaceous Marilyn Monroe.)

I recall sitting in a darkened movie theater looking up at a screen filled with the voluptuous bodies of Marilyn Monroe and Jane Russell singing "Diamonds Are a Girl's Best Friend." Their skintight, figure-revealing costumes made me think that something else was also a girl's best friend!

Compared to these two movie stars, I definitely had major figure problems. My solution: to requisition the piano bench as a workout station and two large cans of fruit juice as hand weights. I worked out to the cadence of "I must, I must, I must increase my bust." It was all to little avail.

Throughout the years I compared my figure to those of movie stars, magazine models, and my friends. I kept looking in my mirror and frowning.

Do you compare your figure to others, and feel negative about yourself?

A 4-F IMAGE

I didn't learn how to smile at my reflection until I was forty, married for the second time, the mother of three, and out of a job due to a recent move to Pittsburgh. I got shocked into doing something about my appearance after I saw a picture that my nephew had taken of me. Did I really look that bad? Had I actually gone out in public looking like that?

Have you ever been surprised at the difference between your photographs and what you see in your mirror?

Although my appearance often earned a frown when I looked in the mirror, I certainly didn't remember looking that awful. Now I looked—really looked—at myself.

I was definitely what I would later call 4-F: forty, fat, faded, and frumpy!

I needed HELP. Immediately. I had a limited budget, but desperation is a big motivator. There were no professional image consultants in Pittsburgh in 1980, so with high hopes, I drove all the way to Washington, D.C., to start my make-over by having my colors charted. That was when I had my second shock.

Jan Larkey, the art teacher who had been teaching color theory to hundreds of students, was wearing all the wrong colors!

Changing my wardrobe colors and getting my first compliments in years gave me the idea of applying my art knowledge of color, shape, emphasis, line, and proportion to my own appearance. I soon felt as if I had emerged from a second cocoon. I knew that I would never again have to feel negative about the way I look. For the first time in my life, I was truly in control of my appearance.

Today I still look in the mirror and smile. No, I don't have a knockout figure now. Even though I struggle daily to resist extra calories and follow a program of regular exercise, I would be happy to have that teen figure back. The curves I've added in the interim years are not all in the places I would have chosen! The reason for my smile: I have learned how to camouflage some of my figure problems, divert attention from the ones I can't hide, and accent my assets.

Do you want to change your appearance but wonder where to start?

Changing the outside of me had a dramatic impact on the inside of me. My confidence soared. My husband, who had been resisting any changes—especially the addition of makeup—soon took delight in my metamorphosis. My elation at becoming the "new, revised, Jan Larkey" prompted me to train as a color consultant so I could share this knowledge with others.

Throughout my early years as a color and image consultant, my clients asked me endless questions about their figures. I discovered that even women with gorgeous bodies were incredibly critical about themselves. They also were confused by fashion terms and by the overwhelming variety of styles available.

For several years I searched for solutions to figure problems. My frustration grew with the stacks of information. In most publications, the few pages devoted to dos and don'ts for figure problems typically considered each problem as if it were the *only* one you might have. The resulting advice was frequently contradictory. For example: If you had short legs, you were advised to wear a shorter jacket to make your legs appear longer. A few pages later, you might be told that if you had a protruding abdomen, you should wear a longer jacket to cover it. Well, what if you had both short legs *and* a protruding abdomen? Which jacket length would flatter you the most? (The answers to this and other questions are found in Chapter 3, where your own unique combination of figure problems will be cross-referenced to more than 250 style illustrations.)

I also tested several conventional figure-typing systems. Most systems used today classify body shape into four prescribed categories with specific characteristics and clever names such as Pear, Athletic, and Rubenesque or initials like *A* or *X*. Others use scientific names such as Ectomorph. While helpful, they typically assess the shape of your body only from the frontal view, without considering whether your pear-shaped figure may also have a long or short neck or whether your ectomorphic form includes a protruding or flat derriere.

I wanted a system that would consider *all* of us—front, side, and back views!

I tried sorting real women's figures into only four standard figure types, but their bodies didn't cooperate. Everyone seemed to have at least two or more characteristics that deviated from the descriptions. Then I tried measuring figures. I made countless trips to a local spa where women of all ages, sizes, and shapes were kind enough to volunteer their figures for me to measure up one side and down the other. I discovered that inches don't tell you how you will look in your clothes. For example: Consider two women with 36-inch bust measurements. One may be "all back" with a very small bust; the other "all bust" with a narrow back! Obviously blouses, dresses, and jackets will look very different on these "same-size" women.

How could figures be evaluated without the limitations of measurements or categories, I wondered. The answer to this dilemma turned out to be both easy and fun. After considerable experimentation, I discovered that by placing two sticks and a string on the body (as illustrated on pages 18–22), women could see their body *proportions* more clearly than ever before.

Proportion considers the size of each body part as it relates to your total body. When one part of your body appears to be too small or too large in comparison to the rest of you, your total image appears unbalanced. This is a figure problem. If you look in the mirror and see hips that look too large, a neck that looks too short, or a bustline like entertainer Dolly Parton's, you are viewing that part of your body in relation to the rest of you.

Body parts are relative. Dolly Parton, for example, is a small woman with a tiny waist and small hips, which she emphasizes with snug-fitting outfits and belts. This makes her ample bustline look even larger by comparison. The same size bosom on a woman who is 5 feet 9 inches and weighs 175 pounds would not be as noticeable because it would be less disproportionate to the rest of her body.

The guidelines in *FYF* consider how *all* of your body parts relate to your total figure. It avoids the confusion of trying to fit your figure into a specific type, the risk of measuring inaccurately, or the mistake of considering only one figure problem at a time. *Flatter Your Figure* focuses on how you look in your clothes, but more important than that, it emphasizes how you *feel* about the way you look in your clothes.

THROUGH THE LOOKING GLASS: MIRRORS AND MOTHERS

How do you feel when you look in your mirror?

Your earliest input about your appearance probably came from your mother. If she was like many mothers, you got conflicting messages. Motherly advice such as "It's not what is on the outside that counts, it's what is on the inside," may have been followed by "Surely you are not going out looking like *that!*" She may have told you, "Beauty is only skin deep," and "Pretty is as pretty does," while continually correcting the way you looked.

A relative of mine summarized her relationship with her mother with these words, "No matter how hard I tried, I never looked pretty enough to please her. Something was always wrong." Her two teenage daughters instantly responded, "That is exactly the way you make us feel!" They cited examples of things she had said to them: "Why don't you wear your white sweater with that outfit? It will look better than the one you have on," and "Let me get the polish remover for you. You don't want to go out with chipped nails." Their mother looked shocked. What she considered to be motherly help and advice, they considered to be criticism. The moral of the story: Frequent criticism combined with few compliments can lead to negative feelings about yourself that last a lifetime. The second moral: It is hard to feel negative toward someone who makes you feel good about yourself. Don't be stingy with compliments. They are fun to give as well as to receive!

THE BODY BEAUTIFUL: YESTERDAY AND TODAY

Social and cultural changes influence our perception of the ideal body. The ideal by which women judge themselves has changed drastically in recent decades.

In the 1950s the figures of international movie queens such as Marilyn Monroe, Brigitte Bardot, and Sophia Loren set the standards of beauty as curves, bosoms, sensuousness, and sexiness. The 1960s and 1970s saw the pendulum swing all the way to the opposite extreme. The back-to-nature hippie movement espoused shapeless garments, no makeup, and long, straight hair. The feminist movement denounced being hired—or judged—on appearance rather than on brains and ability. Beauty contests were picketed. The ugliest object near the Stanford campus, the Bayshore Freeway, was almost elected homecoming queen when I attended college there!

The 1980s brought a rebellion against the rigid dress-for-success formulas of the late 1970s, which had businesswomen dressing like men in tailored suits and white shirts with little ribbon bows. Women also refused, en masse, to buy thigh-high hemlines that exposed a maturing leg. No longer were we going to be consumer slaves to drastic, unflattering dictates of fashion trends.

Simultaneously the fledgling image industry exploded with the publication of Carole Jackson's book *Color Me Beautiful* (Ballantine, 1980). For the first time women were looking in the mirror to see how the color of their clothes related to *them* rather than buying the latest colors, flattering or not. The time to express yourself as an individual had arrived!

Throughout the years, constant comparisons to the tallest, thinnest, youngest, most glamorous women have resulted in drastic actions by some women. Some have chosen to undergo extensive plastic surgery. Others are so upset about being overweight that they develop eating disorders that too often result in permanent health problems or even death.

Today, the pendulum rests in a more moderate and realistic position. While research substantiates that our appearance does make a difference in how others relate to us in both our personal and professional lives, we no longer must feel inferior because we do not measure up to a narrow view of what is beautiful or professional.

The image to aspire to in the 1990s is *healthy:* a healthy body and a healthy attitude toward the body. The most beautiful women of the 1990s will be those whose self-confidence radiates to others because they are making the most of their individual potential. Whether today's woman is making cookies or career choices (or both), she will make the effort each morning to look the best she can look; then she can forget about her appearance and turn her energy toward accomplishing the tasks at hand.

REALITY

For women of the 1990s reality is that 90 percent of us don't—and won't ever—look like models or movie stars.

Let's look at real women. According to the 1987 *Statistical Abstract of the United States Government,* the average American woman is just under 5 feet 4 inches tall, weighs 142 pounds, and is thirty-two years old. Her hips are wider than her shoulders. She is a stocky size 12. It is no wonder that she feels negative about herself when she compares herself to tall, svelte models. The reality is that the fashion industry labels women who are 5 feet 4 inches as petites, when actually that is the height of the *average* woman! When you think about it, tall skinny models are the ones who are "abnormal."

In real life no one is as tall or as thin as mannequins or fashion illustrations. According to Stuart Ewen, author of *All Consuming Images* (Basic Books, 1988), almost every photograph that appears in fashion magazines is retouched. Even the models don't look as good as their own photographs!

Reality is that having a fabulous figure is a temporary condition at best. The sands of time eventually shift even hourglass figures.

Reality is the woman who got out of your bed this morning and recognized that the figure in the mirror may never be rated a perfect 10 or even a size 10. Nevertheless, while clothing cannot make a woman who is 5 feet 4 inches look like she is 5 feet 8 inches or a heavy woman appear 40 pounds thinner, clothing *can* help *every* woman, regardless of her height or weight, receive the ultimate compliment: "You always look so nice."

The ultimate self put-down is to feel negative about your appearance and to do nothing about it. I'm delighted that you have chosen to do something about your appearance today. By reading this book you have made a commitment to yourself to stop hiding your potential and to bring out the best in you.

Looking in your mirror and smiling should be your goal every day regardless of age, size, or shape. As you get dressed, keep in mind: The most important person you need to impress each day is yourself. A positive response to yourself is contagious. When you feel good about yourself, others will, also.

Are you ready to look in your mirror and smile? Great. The next step toward that goal is to have some fun learning how to—"FOoooOF."

CHAPTER
2

"FOoooOF"
(Figuring Out Our Figures)

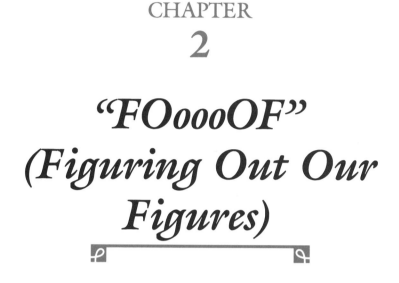

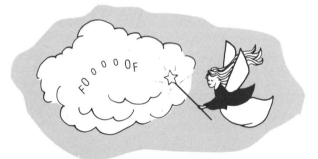

The first step in "figuring out our figures" is to start with the way we see ourselves. Write some brief phrases that describe your body in the space below.

Describe Your Body:_____

_____

_____

I know that some of you are thinking, "I'll read ahead and do that later." What I have learned in working with thousands of women is *that most women do not see themselves as others see them.* How you see yourself is critical in accurately evaluating your figure. Do take just a few moments now to jot down some descriptive words or phrases.

Good. Now read on.

If you are like most of the women at my seminars, you probably focused on your negative features and wrote subjective descriptions such as: short, overweight, big hips, thick ankles. In contrast, I've found that men focus on the facts: 5 foot 10 inches, brown hair, brown eyes. Compare the answers of three female and three male friends when you ask them to describe their bodies.

The second step is to consider what you would like to change about your figure. A Gallup Poll for *American Health Magazine* (1988) found that "today's woman would like to grow another inch taller, drop 2 dress sizes, lose 11 pounds and have a lean muscular body." In 1987, a *Shape* magazine survey reported, "What 9000 women liked least and most wanted to change were their thighs, hips, buttocks, stomach, and waist."

What would you like to change about your figure? If Cinderella's fairy godmother did appear and offered to grant your figure fantasies, where would you want her to point her magic wand?

List any figure challenges you wish you could magically change below, starting with the one that bothers you the most.

Figure Challenges List:_____

_____

_____

Now that you have listed your perceived figure problems, take the following "Image Quotient (I.Q.)" quiz to discover just how objective you have been.

IMAGE QUOTIENT (I.Q.) QUIZ

Complete each statement by *circling the response that describes you best.*

Me and My Image

1. When I see pictures/videos of myself I
   a. am shocked.
   b. am surprised at how I really look.
   c. am pleased with my appearance.
   d. look the way I remember looking on that day.

2. On a scale of 1 to 10 I would rate my figure as
   a. 1–2 terrible.
   b. 3–5 not very attractive.
   c. 6–8 good.
   d. 9–10 terrific.
3. I think my body weight is
   a. 10 to 15 pounds too heavy.
   b. a major problem.
   c. acceptable for my age and height.
   d. not a problem.
4. I have negative thoughts about my body
   a. daily.
   b. often.
   c. occasionally.
   d. rarely.
5. I make an effort to look my best
   a. for special occasions only.
   b. when I can find the time.
   c. most days.
   d. every day.
6. Compared to five years ago my figure is
   a. hopeless.
   b. worse.
   c. about the same.
   d. better.
7. The first thing I look at in a full-length mirror is
   a. one of my figure problems.
   b. nothing, because I avoid looking in mirrors.
   c. my overall appearance.
   d. my best features.

Others and My Image

8. I receive compliments about my appearance
   a. almost never.
   b. rarely.
   c. when I get dressed up.
   d. frequently.
9. When I receive a compliment I
   a. really don't believe it.
   b. discount it with a negative comment (such as, "I need to lose more").
   c. feel wonderful.
   d. say thank you.

10. When casually dressed at home and my doorbell rings unexpectedly, I am most likely to
    a. panic and not answer it.
    b. answer it and apologize about the way I look.
    c. answer it without worrying because I usually look fine.
    d. make a quick attempt to look better and then answer it.
11. When I was growing up, my parents reacted to my appearance this way:
    a. My mother was critical, my father rarely commented.
    b. No one seemed to care how I looked.
    c. My mother was positive.
    d. Both my parents were positive.

Shopping to Create My Image

12. Before purchasing clothing I often ask the opinion of
    a. friends or family.
    b. salespeople or strangers.
    c. just myself.
    d. I ask others, but I purchase only the items I think look good on me.
13. After shopping, I
    a. wonder why I bought something.
    b. often return things.
    c. can't wait to wear my new clothes.
    d. have fun combining the new items with my other clothes.
14. Before deciding to purchase a garment, I
    a. look at the merchandise in several stores.
    b. try on four or more other garments.
    c. try on three garments or less.
    d. buy something immediately if it is what I need.

Total of all of your *a* and *b* answers_____
Total of all of your *c* and *d* answers_____

If you have eleven or more *c* and *d* answers, you have an overall positive, healthy body image and see yourself objectively enough to do the figure analysis in this chapter with the assistance of one friend. If you have four or more *a* and *b* answers, ask two or more friends to help you evaluate your figure accurately and objectively. The more *a* and *b* answers you have—the more friends you should call! The more, the merrier. Besides providing more objective opinions, "FOoooOF-ing" together is fun. Enjoy sharing the laughter and warmth that occur when a group of friends kick off their shoes and use two sticks and a string to figure out their figures.

Be prepared to find out that you and your friends are probably too critical of yourselves. You may find yourself telling them that you never even noticed something that they think is awful about their body, and you will probably hear the same thing from them! You may be in for an eye-opening experience when you learn to see yourself as others see you.

Assistance is also available from professionals familiar with the *Flatter Your Figure* system. Send the request form in the back of this book for the name of your nearest professional or school offering classes and programs based on *FYF*.

Why is it so hard to see yourself accurately? Because the reflection you see in the mirror is clouded by all your memories, experiences, and past comments about your figure. Comments from your parents (question 11) turn out to be important in the development of positive or negative feelings about yourself. Answer *a* is the one most often experienced by women with low self-esteem.

WHEN IS A FIGURE PROBLEM NOT A FIGURE PROBLEM?

If you are still thinking of evaluating your own figure by yourself, consider what would have happened if the following women had done so.

In *FYF* classes, the participants form groups to help each other do the stick-and-string tests on pages 18–22 while the instructor circulates, assisting as needed. During one class, a lovely woman of about thirty came up to me in a huff. "My group just told me that I *don't* have a hip problem!" Looking at her slim hips, I asked what problem she thought she had. Her answer: "I have trouble finding clothes that fit because I am a size 6 on the bottom and an 8 on the top." With a smile I explained that having smaller hips than shoulders is considered an asset, not a problem. She had a *fit problem,* not a figure problem.

A few minutes later she was back. "Now they tell me that my shoulders don't slump!" she exclaimed. I checked the alignment of her shoulders and reported that her group was right. "Oh, but they can't be. My mother has told me all of my life to sit up straight." I suggested that she tell her mother that her warnings had worked, because her posture was terrific.

Several weeks later when I happened to see her, she reported that her mother was very upset with me for saying that she did not have a shoulder problem. That's when it became obvious that while this lovely young woman did not have a figure problem—she did have a *mother problem!*

One of the largest sewing-machine companies in the United States invited me to conduct a *FYF* workshop for their educational department. As we were concluding the sticks and string tests, the department head expressed surprise, "I always thought that I was long waisted." I double-checked her waist placement and assured her that her waist length was average. "Then why do I always need to add 2 inches to the bodice of patterns to make them long enough?" she asked. I asked her how tall she was. Her answer was 5 feet, 9 inches. "That," I replied, "is 5 inches taller than the average woman's height. Just because you need to add to a pattern does not mean that you have a figure problem. It just means that patterns are not scaled to your height." An *alteration problem* on a pattern or garment does not necessarily mean that you have a figure problem.

Without assistance in figuring out their figures, these women would have erroneously marked flattering styles throughout this workbook as being unflattering! If you have any doubts about identifying your figure problems correctly, please get assistance from friends or professionals. I don't want you to go even one more day thinking you have figure problems if what you really have are *fit, alteration—or mother— problems.*

WHAT'S THE PROBLEM?

FIT PROBLEM.   Fit refers to the size and shape of the garment in relation to the size and shape of your body. Telltale signs of a poor fit are binding across the shoulders, bosom, or hips or bunching of excess fabric in an area.

Note: Just because a garment fits your body doesn't automatically mean that the style is flattering. For example, the design lines of a fantastically fitted outfit may make you look heavier or call attention to a figure problem.

ALTERATION PROBLEM.   Ready-to-wear clothing or standardized patterns may need alterations, such as longer sleeves or pant legs, to adjust to your size or shape. Just because a garment needs to be altered does not mean that you have a figure problem.

WEIGHT PROBLEM.   Being overweight is a concern for many women even if they have perfect proportions. A special section titled Dressing Thinner has been included in Chapter 4 to help you create slimming illusions with clothing.

SIZE PROBLEM. Manufacturers and pattern companies do not label all sizes exactly the same way. Size tags are only estimates of what will possibly fit. Generally, expensive garments are cut more generously and fit with more ease than lower-priced items that are cut to minimize fabric usage. Regardless of the label, your mirror should be your guide to the right size. It is the number of compliments you get when wearing an outfit, not the numbers on the tag, that really count!

MOTHER/OTHER PROBLEM. Criticism or misunderstood statements from others can create a false image of your body. Don't let yesterday's negative memories keep you from accepting the objective opinions of the supportive friends who are helping you today. Five pairs of friendly eyes won't be wrong!

MINOR FIGURE PROBLEM. A problem that does not distract the viewer's attention from seeing your overall appearance is Minor.

MAJOR FIGURE PROBLEM. This is a problem that is easily seen by others. It detracts from your overall appearance. A problem becomes Major whenever a viewer's attention is drawn to it.

IMAGINARY PROBLEM. This is a problem you think you have that no one else can see. (Don't be surprised if you have to give up one of your "favorite" figure problems!)

DETERMINING MAJOR VS. MINOR FIGURE PROBLEMS

There are nineteen illustrated figure problems on the following pages interspersed with the stick-and-string figure assessments. The first five problems concern your total body proportions. Problems six through nineteen focus on specific parts of your figure. You will not find long or short arms on the list of figure problems. Why? Think about what you visually notice about other people. How many times have you looked at a woman and thought, "Goodness, she has long arms!" Probably rarely, if ever. *FYF* focuses on camouflaging the problems that visually detract from your appearance.

Most women have between three and seven figure problems. Some of these are minor. A Minor figure problem is noticed mainly by you. It is *not* as obvious as the problem drawn in the illustration. For example: Your upper arm isn't as firm as it used to be. Don't compare today's body with the body you used to have. Instead, *use the drawings as your basis of comparison in determining if your problem is Minor or Major.* A Major figure problem is a problem without any doubt. It is easily seen by others and definitely resembles the illustrations of the Major problems.

Be aware that in doing self-analysis you may succumb to the tendency to see every minor figure problem as a major one. I call that the "Pinocchio's Nose Syndrome"—the more you focus on it in the mirror, the bigger it gets! That's why it's so important to compare your body to the illustrations.

When in doubt and when your friends can't decide if your problem is Major or Minor—it is Minor.

READY? TIME TO HAVE SOME FUN "FOoooOF-ing"

You need:

1. Two sticks. These may be curtain rods or dowel rods. You may use the edges of yardsticks *only* if you resist the temptation to measure anything!
2. One string, at least 4 feet long (a sash, belt, or ribbon will do).
3. A friendly helper. A full-length mirror is needed if you have only one helper.
4. A pencil, not a pen—figure problems can change!

Note: No leotard or special clothing is required as you will be able to do the following figure analysis in regular garments.

INSTRUCTIONS FOR HELPERS

Please be just as honest in analyzing others' figures as you would want them to be with you. To pretend that someone doesn't have a figure problem will keep them from learning how to solve it. The most helpful friend is the one who says, "Yes, I can see that problem. It looks like the problem in the illustrations. It needs to be circled as a Major (or Minor) problem so that you can learn how to camouflage it." Before starting, please review the sections above on figure problems.

THE STICK-AND-STRING PROPORTIONAL TESTS

The following stick-and-string tests allow you to see your proportions: how the size of one part of your figure *visually* relates to the rest of you.

I know it will be tempting to measure some things, especially if you are a seamstress. Forget about inches! Measurements are for fitting garments, *not* for figuring out which patterns will look good on you.

HOW TO MARK YOUR FIGURE PROBLEMS

No Apparent Problem: Great! Proceed to the next figure problem.

Minor Problems: If your problem is *not* as noticeable as the one shown in the illustration, circle "MINOR." Example:

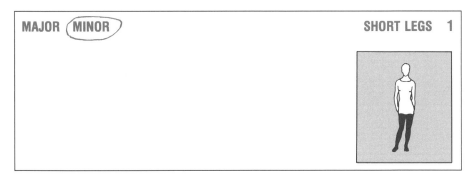

MAJOR (MINOR)

SHORT LEGS 1

Major Problems: If your problem is as obvious as the one shown in the illustration, circle "MAJOR."

Undecided? If in doubt, it is a MINOR problem!

The **goals** and **tips** with each figure problem provide guidelines for solving Minor problems. Solutions for Major problems are illustrated in Chapter 3.

COMPARE YOUR BODY TO THE ILLUSTRATIONS—NOT TO MODELS, MOVIE STARS, OR MANNEQUINS OR THE WAY YOUR BODY LOOKED WHEN YOU WERE YOUNGER.

TEST I. ARE YOUR LEGS AND YOUR TORSO VISUALLY BALANCED?

A positive proportion occurs when your legs appear to be as long as, or longer than, the top of your body (torso plus head).

Model and helper: Stand 5 or more feet from the mirror or group, so that the test results can be accurately observed. The model should remove her shoes.

1. *Model:* Face the mirror or group.
2. *Helper:* Have the model hold one stick across the top of her legs at the leg-hip crease (use both hands). To check placement: have her bend slightly at the hips, then stand up straight.
3. *Helper:* Place the second stick across the top of her head *parallel* to her shoulders as illustrated. **Compare the body lengths above and below the leg-length stick to the illustrations** and follow the directions for marking any figure problem.

A. SHORT LEGS

Legs *slightly* shorter:
   Circle the word MINOR for Figure Problem #1 SHORT LEGS, illustrated below.
Legs *distinctly* shorter than the rest of the body:
   Circle the word MAJOR for Figure Problem #1 SHORT LEGS.

B. VISUALLY BALANCED

No figure problem.
Long legs are an asset, not a problem.

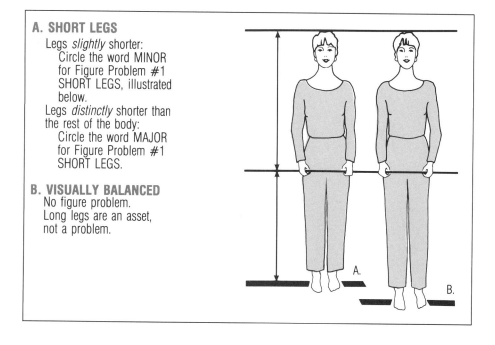

A.

B.

MAJOR   MINOR
Do Proportional Test I.

SHORT LEGS   1

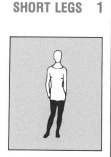

Short legs are a problem for the majority of women.

Goal: To lengthen legs visually.

Tips: Wear garments with vertical lines from the waist down, such as pleats, seams, rows of buttons, or pants with creases. Wear one color from waist to toe. Refer to your best skirt, pant, and jacket lengths (pages 45 and 47) for hemming garments.

Petite Tip

When is a Petite not a Petite? If you are almost 5 feet 4 inches and your legs are distinctly shorter than the rest of you, you are probably a "Misses" with short legs! Shop at both Misses and Petite stores.

TEST II. DO YOUR HIPS AND SHOULDERS VISUALLY BALANCE?

Ideally, your shoulders should appear to be as wide as, or slightly wider than, your hips.

1. *Model:* Face the mirror or group; clasp your hands behind your back.

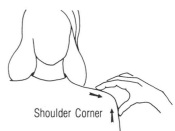

Shoulder Corner

2. *Helper:* Find her shoulder "corner" (where the shoulder and arm meet) by sliding your finger and thumb together as illustrated. (Feel *under* shoulder pads.)

3. Place one end of the stick at the shoulder corner in *front* of her arm as illustrated. Allow the other end of the stick to touch the widest part of the hip/thigh area. *Observe the angle of the stick* and follow the instructions under the appropriate illustration.

Note: A Protruding Abdomen or Derriere may add to a "bottom-heavy" image. Heavy Arms and/or a Full Bust add to a "top-heavy" look. These problems are addressed later. For now, look at the angle of the stick and consider only the widths of the hip and shoulder.

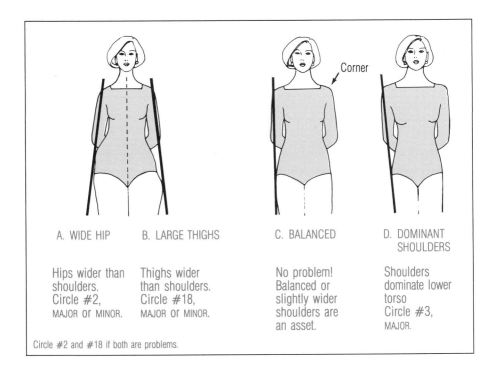

A. WIDE HIP	B. LARGE THIGHS	C. BALANCED	D. DOMINANT SHOULDERS
Hips wider than shoulders. Circle #2, MAJOR or MINOR.	Thighs wider than shoulders. Circle #18, MAJOR or MINOR.	No problem! Balanced or slightly wider shoulders are an asset.	Shoulders dominate lower torso Circle #3, MAJOR.

Circle #2 and #18 if both are problems.

MAJOR   MINOR

Do Proportional Test II.

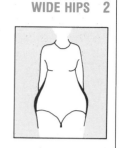

WIDE HIPS   2

Goal: To widen the shoulders to visually balance the hips.
Tips: Add shoulder pads to everything (if you are considerably overweight, use small pads). Vertical lines from the waist down will slim hips. Horizontal lines on the upper torso will widen shoulders. Add volume above the waist.

MAJOR

Do Proportional Test II.

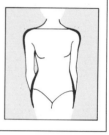

DOMINANT SHOULDERS   3

Note: *Slightly* wider shoulders are an asset.
Goal: To narrow shoulders.
Tips: Wear open necklines, vertical stripes or tucks. Avoid bulky fabrics, large shoulder pads, and horizontal lines in the shoulder area. Add fullness to lower garments only if hips are slim.

TEST III. ARE YOU LONG- OR SHORT-WAISTED?

Your torso is visually divided into upper and lower torso by a waistline. Ideally *you should be slightly longer above your waist.*

Note: Some women look short-waisted from the front when they are really just low-bosomed!

1. *Model:* Tie the string around your natural waistline. *Check the side view first* before using the sticks. If the string looks almost level from the side view, proceed to step 2. If the string looks like either of these drawings, follow the guidelines beside them.

A. If the angle of the string goes up in the front, circle #4 Short Waisted, MAJOR.
Evaluate #8 Round Shoulders and #16 Flat Derriere now.

B. If the angle of the string goes up in the back, circle #5 Long Waisted, MAJOR.
Evaluate #15, Protruding Derriere or Swaybacked now.

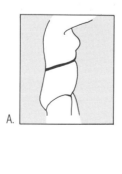

2. *Model:* Turn your back to the mirror or group, and hold the stick behind your back at the top of your legs (under the curve of your hips) as if you are "sitting" on it. This defines the torso length.

3. *Helper:* Place the second stick straight across her shoulders from corner to corner as illustrated. Compare the length of the torso above and below the string to the illustrations.

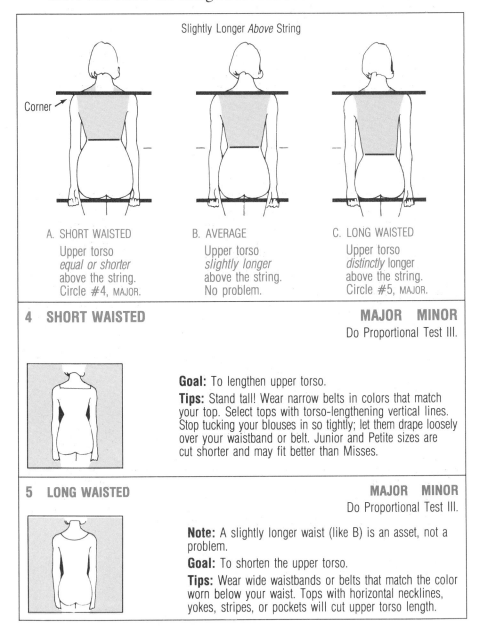

Slightly Longer *Above* String

Corner ➤

A. SHORT WAISTED
Upper torso *equal or shorter* above the string. Circle #4, MAJOR.

B. AVERAGE
Upper torso *slightly longer* above the string. No problem.

C. LONG WAISTED
Upper torso *distinctly* longer above the string. Circle #5, MAJOR.

4 SHORT WAISTED　　　　　　　　　　　**MAJOR   MINOR**
Do Proportional Test III.

Goal: To lengthen upper torso.

Tips: Stand tall! Wear narrow belts in colors that match your top. Select tops with torso-lengthening vertical lines. Stop tucking your blouses in so tightly; let them drape loosely over your waistband or belt. Junior and Petite sizes are cut shorter and may fit better than Misses.

5 LONG WAISTED　　　　　　　　　　　**MAJOR   MINOR**
Do Proportional Test III.

Note: A slightly longer waist (like B) is an asset, not a problem.

Goal: To shorten the upper torso.

Tips: Wear wide waistbands or belts that match the color worn below your waist. Tops with horizontal necklines, yokes, stripes, or pockets will cut upper torso length.

Complete your figure analysis by comparing your body to the illustrations.

MAJOR   MINOR   **SHORT NECK and/or DOUBLE CHIN   6**

Compare to the drawings.

Goal: To visually elongate or thin your neck.

Tips: Wear necklines open or below the collarbone. Hairstyles up or off the neck are flattering. Avoid short necklaces and high closed collars.

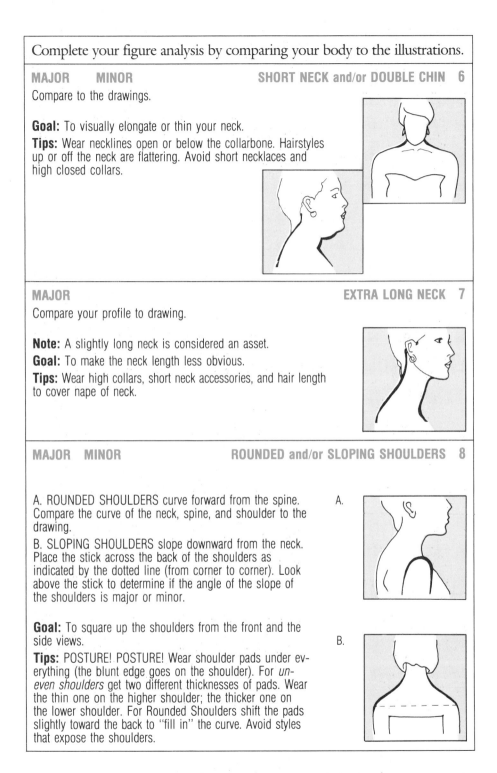

MAJOR   **EXTRA LONG NECK   7**

Compare your profile to drawing.

Note: A slightly long neck is considered an asset.

Goal: To make the neck length less obvious.

Tips: Wear high collars, short neck accessories, and hair length to cover nape of neck.

MAJOR   MINOR   **ROUNDED and/or SLOPING SHOULDERS   8**

A. ROUNDED SHOULDERS curve forward from the spine. Compare the curve of the neck, spine, and shoulder to the drawing.

B. SLOPING SHOULDERS slope downward from the neck. Place the stick across the back of the shoulders as indicated by the dotted line (from corner to corner). Look above the stick to determine if the angle of the slope of the shoulders is major or minor.

Goal: To square up the shoulders from the front and the side views.

Tips: POSTURE! POSTURE! Wear shoulder pads under everything (the blunt edge goes on the shoulder). For *uneven shoulders* get two different thicknesses of pads. Wear the thin one on the higher shoulder; the thicker one on the lower shoulder. For Rounded Shoulders shift the pads slightly toward the back to "fill in" the curve. Avoid styles that expose the shoulders.

A.

B.

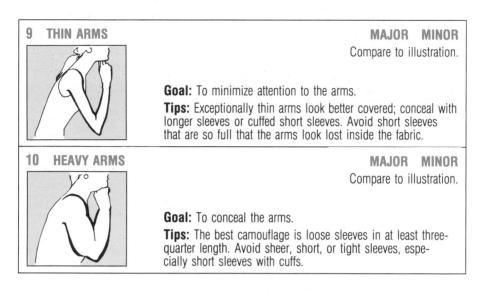

9   THIN ARMS

MAJOR   MINOR
Compare to illustration.

Goal: To minimize attention to the arms.

Tips: Exceptionally thin arms look better covered; conceal with longer sleeves or cuffed short sleeves. Avoid short sleeves that are so full that the arms look lost inside the fabric.

10   HEAVY ARMS

MAJOR   MINOR
Compare to illustration.

Goal: To conceal the arms.

Tips: The best camouflage is loose sleeves in at least three-quarter length. Avoid sheer, short, or tight sleeves, especially short sleeves with cuffs.

BUSTLINE: FULL OR SMALL?

I was surprised to see that a reporter who had marked her own workbook prior to interviewing me had marked Full Bust as one of her Major problems. I had never noticed her bosom. When asked why she thought it was a Major problem, she said, "Because I wear a 38-D bra." While she had just lost 25 pounds, her 38-D bosom was in wonderful proportion to the rest of her 5-foot, 9-inch and 160-pound body. A smaller bosom would have been a figure problem!

Forget your bra size and compare the size of your bosom to the rest of you. Is your bosom proportionally so large or small that it detracts from your appearance? If so, then you can circle MAJOR for Full or Small Bust.

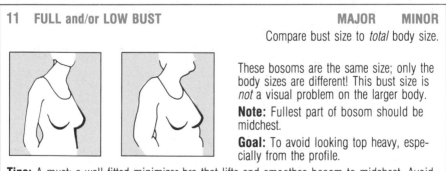

11   FULL and/or LOW BUST

MAJOR   MINOR
Compare bust size to *total* body size.

These bosoms are the same size; only the body sizes are different! This bust size is *not* a visual problem on the larger body.

Note: Fullest part of bosom should be midchest.

Goal: To avoid looking top heavy, especially from the profile.

Tips: A must: a well-fitted minimizer bra that lifts and smoothes bosom to midchest. Avoid rounding your shoulders and creating more figure problems. Avoid wide waistbands or belts that shorten the torso.

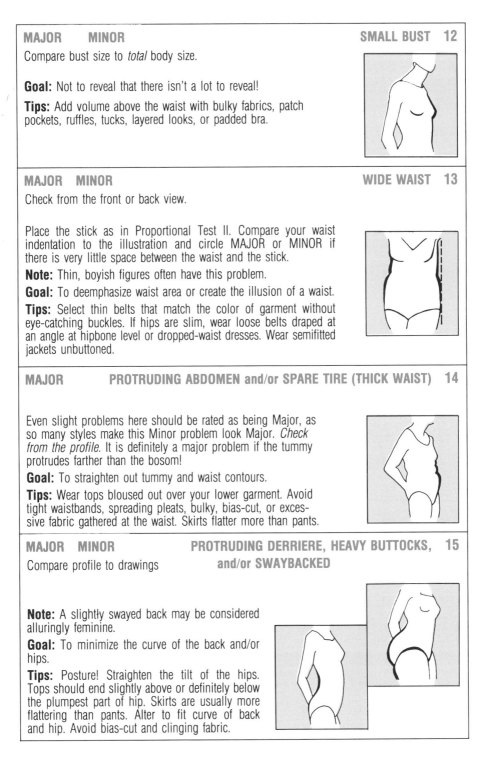

MAJOR   MINOR　　　　　　　　　　　　　　　　　**SMALL BUST   12**

Compare bust size to *total* body size.

Goal: Not to reveal that there isn't a lot to reveal!

Tips: Add volume above the waist with bulky fabrics, patch pockets, ruffles, tucks, layered looks, or padded bra.

MAJOR   MINOR　　　　　　　　　　　　　　　　　**WIDE WAIST   13**

Check from the front or back view.

Place the stick as in Proportional Test II. Compare your waist indentation to the illustration and circle MAJOR or MINOR if there is very little space between the waist and the stick.

Note: Thin, boyish figures often have this problem.

Goal: To deemphasize waist area or create the illusion of a waist.

Tips: Select thin belts that match the color of garment without eye-catching buckles. If hips are slim, wear loose belts draped at an angle at hipbone level or dropped-waist dresses. Wear semifitted jackets unbuttoned.

MAJOR　　　　　**PROTRUDING ABDOMEN and/or SPARE TIRE (THICK WAIST)   14**

Even slight problems here should be rated as being Major, as so many styles make this Minor problem look Major. *Check from the profile.* It is definitely a major problem if the tummy protrudes farther than the bosom!

Goal: To straighten out tummy and waist contours.

Tips: Wear tops bloused out over your lower garment. Avoid tight waistbands, spreading pleats, bulky, bias-cut, or excessive fabric gathered at the waist. Skirts flatter more than pants.

MAJOR   MINOR　　　　　**PROTRUDING DERRIERE, HEAVY BUTTOCKS,   15**
Compare profile to drawings　　　　　　**and/or SWAYBACKED**

Note: A slightly swayed back may be considered alluringly feminine.

Goal: To minimize the curve of the back and/or hips.

Tips: Posture! Straighten the tilt of the hips. Tops should end slightly above or definitely below the plumpest part of hip. Skirts are usually more flattering than pants. Alter to fit curve of back and hip. Avoid bias-cut and clinging fabric.

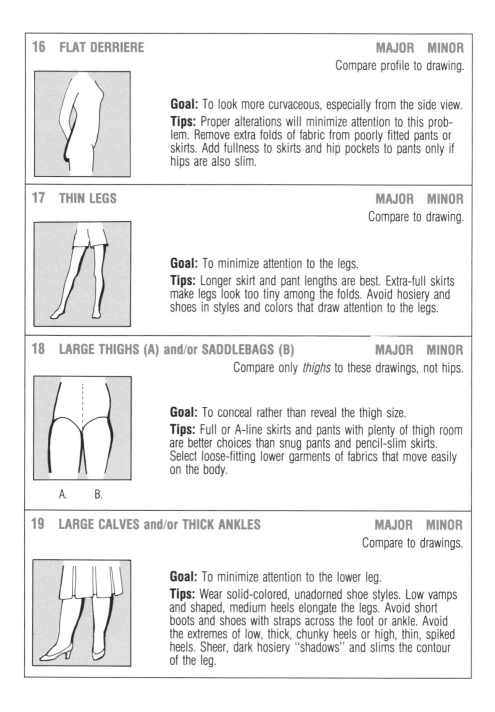

16 FLAT DERRIERE

MAJOR MINOR

Compare profile to drawing.

Goal: To look more curvaceous, especially from the side view.

Tips: Proper alterations will minimize attention to this problem. Remove extra folds of fabric from poorly fitted pants or skirts. Add fullness to skirts and hip pockets to pants only if hips are also slim.

17 THIN LEGS

MAJOR MINOR

Compare to drawing.

Goal: To minimize attention to the legs.

Tips: Longer skirt and pant lengths are best. Extra-full skirts make legs look too tiny among the folds. Avoid hosiery and shoes in styles and colors that draw attention to the legs.

18 LARGE THIGHS (A) and/or SADDLEBAGS (B)

MAJOR MINOR

Compare only *thighs* to these drawings, not hips.

Goal: To conceal rather than reveal the thigh size.

Tips: Full or A-line skirts and pants with plenty of thigh room are better choices than snug pants and pencil-slim skirts. Select loose-fitting lower garments of fabrics that move easily on the body.

A.   B.

19 LARGE CALVES and/or THICK ANKLES

MAJOR MINOR

Compare to drawings.

Goal: To minimize attention to the lower leg.

Tips: Wear solid-colored, unadorned shoe styles. Low vamps and shaped, medium heels elongate the legs. Avoid short boots and shoes with straps across the foot or ankle. Avoid the extremes of low, thick, chunky heels or high, thin, spiked heels. Sheer, dark hosiery "shadows" and slims the contour of the leg.

MARKING YOUR WORKBOOK

MINOR FIGURE PROBLEMS: Study and follow the tips written beside them. Do *not* circle the numbers for Minor problems on the foldout flap or under the style illustrations in the next chapter. To do so will limit too many styles that will be acceptable and attractive on your figure.

MAJOR FIGURE PROBLEM LIST: Fold out the flap on the inside of the cover. Review all nineteen figure problems starting on page 19 and *circle only the numbers of your MAJOR problems* on the list on the flap.

Note: Use a pencil. Figure problems do change, especially during childbearing years and with major weight changes. If you add or lose a figure problem, just adjust your workbook accordingly.

YOUR PERSONAL FIGURE CHART

Inside the back cover is a Figure Chart that, when completed, will be a quick guide to help you select a flattering wardrobe. Refer to the MAJOR figure problems you have just circled on the cover flap and complete the section titled "(-) Figure Problems (-)" now.

Great! Now that you have identified your figure problems correctly and know how to "FOoooOF," the next step is to figure out how clothing can help—or hinder—your appearance.

CHAPTER

3

Figuring Out Fashions

MODELS, MANNEQUINS, AND YOU

While shopping one day I overheard a disappointed voice say, "I just don't see anything here that will work on my figure." I turned, expecting to see a woman with major figure problems. Instead, to my surprise, the speaker was very tall, slender, and well proportioned.

As I looked through the racks, I thought, "The selection here is excellent. Not only is there a variety of colors, but there is also a wonderful diversity of styles." I saw numerous garments that would have enhanced her figure. How sad. This shopper not only walked past many potential purchases, but the salesperson helping her did not even make suggestions.

Do you pass up flattering garments and end up taking all the wrong things to the dressing room?

Have you ever felt "dressing room despair"?

How do you decide what styles to try on?

The merchants of fashion use ultrachic models to tempt you to try the latest trends. As you flip through the pages in a fashion or pattern catalog or watch models float down a runway, you may be thinking,

"Sure, that looks great on that tall, skinny model, but how will it look on *me*? Why don't they use real women for models?" Some magazines are starting to use petite, full-figured, and mature models. There are even new mannequins being designed with an over-forty look. Even so it would be impossible to show every style on every size and shape of figure. If they did use a figure like yours, then your best friend would be upset because they didn't use one like hers.

Despair no more. By the time you complete this chapter, you will know how to look at garments on tall, skinny models and mannequins, or even hanging limply on display hangers, and know which ones to take to the dressing room. The goal: A dressing room (and closet) filled with fabulously flattering clothing.

✸ **It does not matter how a garment is displayed or modeled if you know how to analyze it and assess how it will look on you.**

UNDERSTANDING CLOTHING CONTOURS VS. YOUR CONTOURS

Your body has a distinctive shape; clothing does too. In the previous chapter you discovered how to analyze your figure. This chapter will show you how to analyze clothing by its shape, lines, and length.

Style Shapes

Study the row of silhouettes below to see how fashion trends since the 1920s have created many different shapes.

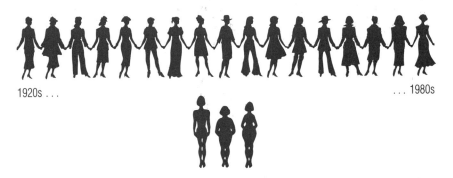

1920s 1980s

Now study the three figure shapes. Select three styles and mentally try them on all three figures. (Aren't you glad that *FYF* avoids categorizing your body into only three or four prescribed shapes? Your figure probably isn't exactly like any of these three silhouettes.)

As you can see, not every garment shape will work on all three figure shapes. Yet each figure can wear a variety of styles that create different silhouettes. So can you. Study the model shown in the following three styles. Notice how her figure takes on a very different shape in each one.

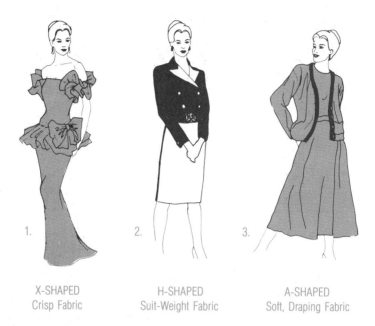

1.	2.	3.
X-SHAPED	H-SHAPED	A-SHAPED
Crisp Fabric	Suit-Weight Fabric	Soft, Draping Fabric

Her figure contours are the same inside each outfit, but the clothing certainly makes them look different. Notice how the different fabrics help to change the silhouette shape.

Style Lines

Within the basic shape/silhouette of each garment are details created by the *lines* of the style. Style lines may be created by seams, tucks, appliqués, pleats, rows of buttons, lapels, and all waistbands and hemlines. The four basic style line directions are horizontal, vertical, diagonal, and curved.

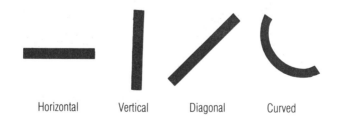

| Horizontal | Vertical | Diagonal | Curved |

Understanding the relationship between the lines of a garment and the shape of your body will help you create flattering illusions. Consider the following rectangles.

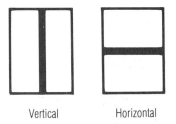

Vertical   Horizontal

Both rectangles are exactly the same size. Notice, however, that the one with the vertical line appears taller; while the one with the horizontal line looks wider.

★ **CONCEPT: The eye looks in the direction of lines: Horizontal lines make you look across; vertical lines make you look up and down.**

Let's translate this concept to clothing lines. Observe how different a figure can look just by how a jacket is worn. In the drawings below, when the jacket is worn open (A), it creates two vertical lines that make you look up and down the body. When the jacket is closed (B), your eye follows the horizontal hemline across the body—especially if the jacket and skirt are different colors.

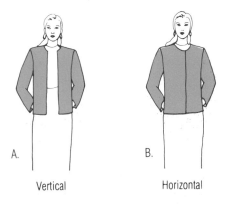

A.   B.

Vertical   Horizontal

★ **CONCEPT: Wear vertical lines on the parts of your body that you want to lengthen or narrow.**

★ **CONCEPT: Wear horizontal lines on the parts of your body that you want to widen or shorten.**

Note: When two or more vertical lines are close together (1, below), they slenderize the figure. If the lines are far apart (2), the eye notices the width of the space between the lines; thus, widely spaced vertical lines can make you look wider!

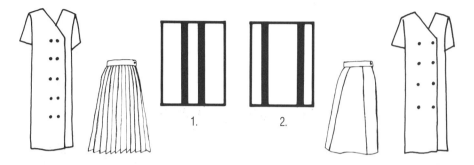

CONVERGING VS. DIVERGING LINES

When diagonal lines come toward each other they *converge*. As they spread apart they *diverge*. Look at the jacket illustrations below and compare how the angle of the lapels changes the illusion of wider hips. (A) or wider shoulders (B).

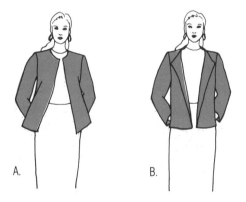

★ CONCEPT: Wear lines that diverge (spread apart) on the parts of your body that you want to look wider. Wear lines that converge (come together) on the parts of your body that you want to look smaller.

★ CONCEPT: When lines converge, they focus attention toward the point where they meet.

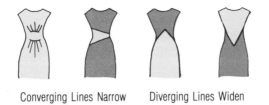

Converging Lines Narrow   Diverging Lines Widen

Diagonal Lines

Diagonal lines go across your body at an angle. The more vertical a diagonal line is, the taller and slimmer you will look. The more horizontal the angle is, the wider you will look.

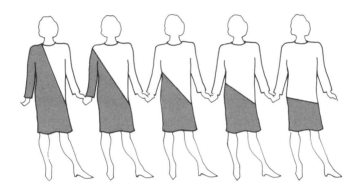

Curved Lines

Curved lines are very feminine and may enhance many figures and faces.

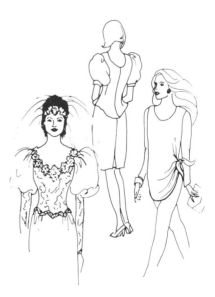

If, however, you feel too curvaceous, be aware of this concept: **Repeating a shape will emphasize it.** Compare these two face shapes. They are exactly the same width. (If you doubt it, measure them!)

FACE SHAPES

A. Full bangs create horizontal lines that widen and shorten the face. Excessive hair at the widest part of the face adds volume. The repetition of a round neckline, round beads, and a round face makes her face look fuller.

B. Notice how hair that is flatter on the sides creates a vertical shape that thins the face. Half-bangs and fullness at the crown create height. The longer, angular necklace creates a V-shape that is more noticeable than the round neckline and adds to the illusion of a longer, slimmer face.

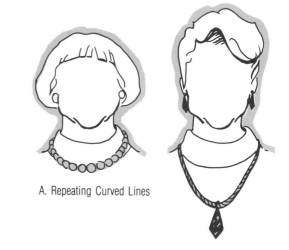

A. Repeating Curved Lines

B. Creating Illusions

Style Lengths

Hemlines and waistlines are horizontal lines. Their length and position can dramatically change the visual proportions of your upper and lower body. You can create the illusion of a longer torso or legs just by changing the length of your tops or waistlines.

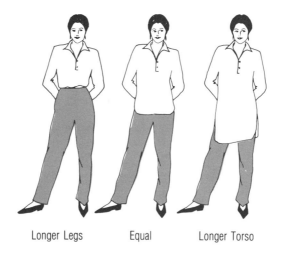

Longer Legs   Equal   Longer Torso

Notice how visual interest is increased when the horizontal line is higher or lower on the figure rather than halfway in-between.

Tip: Avoid placing *obvious* horizontal lines on the widest part of your anatomy! To minimize the impact of a less-than-flattering horizontal line, wear tops and bottoms that are the same or similar colors.

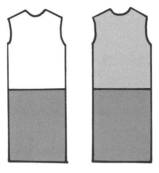

Maximizes Line   Minimizes Line

Length vs. Width

Compare the skirt silhouettes below to see how the length and fullness of garments affect how wide your body appears in comparison to your height.

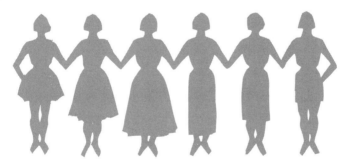

Tip: To look taller and slimmer, wear skirts that appear longer than they are wide.

A STYLE GUIDE THAT TAKES THE GUESSWORK OUT OF SHOPPING

To help you understand how line and design concepts work on your own figure, the following pages of styles have been analyzed for you. Your figure problems have been cross-referenced to hundreds of style illustrations so that you can tell at a glance if a particular garment will flatter your *entire* figure. While many of the styles illustrated in the Style Guide are fashionable now, others will become "fashion forward" again in the future. *FYF* will be a great shopping reference for you year after year.

HOW TO PERSONALIZE THE STYLE GUIDE

1. *Fold out the flap on the cover.* Refer to the Major figure problem numbers you circled at the conclusion of the last chapter.
2. Go through the entire Style Guide and *circle your figure problem numbers wherever they appear under each style illustration.* Each style may have more than one number circled.
3. *Circle all the tips in this chapter that refer to your Figure problem numbers.*

Do not circle Minor problem numbers. Study the goals and tips in the previous chapter for guidelines for solving minor problems.

As you circle your numbers, you will notice that there are two rows of numbers under each illustration: One marked plus (+), the other minus (-). Don't worry about what they mean; just circle all of your numbers wherever they appear. You will learn how to interpret the results later in this chapter.

If you discover that you have only minor problems (it happens), count your blessings and smile more. Do scan the rest of this chapter before proceeding to the next one to learn how to maximize your assets.

Circle all of your Major figure problem numbers on the following pages now.

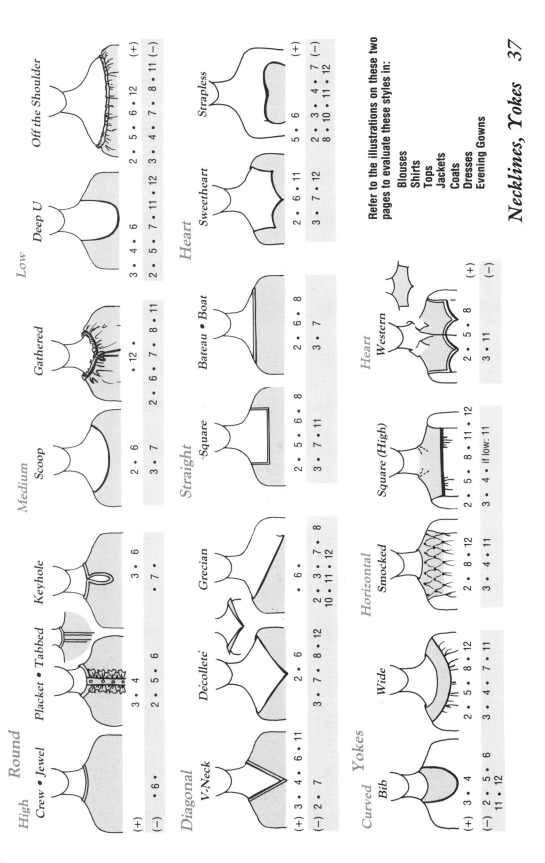

Necklines, Yokes

High Round

Crew • Jewel
(+) • 6 •
(−) 2 • 7

Placket • Tabbed
3 • 4
2 • 5 • 6

Keyhole
3 • 6
• 7 •

Medium

Scoop
2 • 6
3 • 7

Gathered
• 12 •
2 • 6 • 7 • 8 • 11

Low

Deep U
3 • 4 • 6
2 • 5 • 7 • 11 • 12

Off the Shoulder
2 • 5 • 6 • 12
3 • 4 • 7 • 8 • 11 (−)
(+)

Diagonal

V-Neck
(+) 3 • 4 • 6 • 11
(−) 2 • 7

Décolleté
2 • 6
3 • 7 • 8 • 12

Grecian
• 6 •
2 • 3 • 7 •
10 • 11 • 12

Straight

Square
2 • 5 • 6 • 8
3 • 7 • 11

Bateau • Boat
2 • 6 • 8
3 • 7

Heart

Sweetheart
2 • 6 • 11
3 • 7 • 12

Strapless
5 • 6
2 • 3 • 4 • 7 •
8 • 10 • 11 • 12

Refer to the illustrations on these two pages to evaluate these styles in:

**Blouses
Shirts
Tops
Jackets
Coats
Dresses
Evening Gowns**

Yokes

Curved

Bib
(+) 3 • 4
(−) 2 • 5 • 6
11 • 12

Wide
2 • 5 • 8 • 12
3 • 4 • 7 • 11

Horizontal

Smocked
2 • 8 • 12
3 • 4 • 11

Square (High)
2 • 5 • 8 • 11 • 12
3 • 4 • if low: 11

Heart

Western
2 • 5 • 8
3 • 11
(+)
(−)

37

Collars, Lapels 38

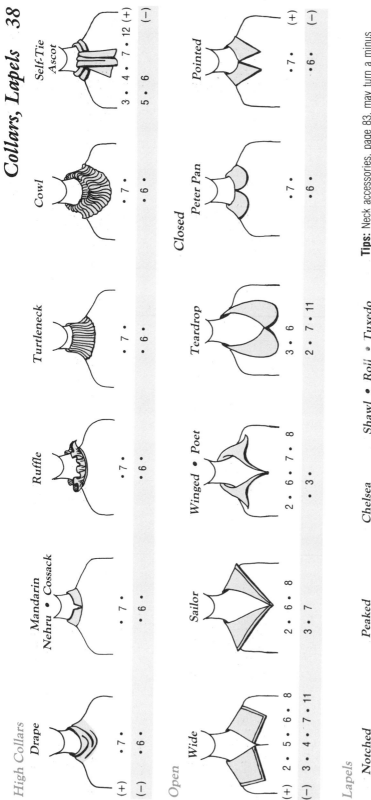

High Collars

Drape
(+) • 7 •
(−) • 6 •

Mandarin
Nehru • Cossack
• 7 •
• 6 •

Ruffle
• 7 •
• 6 •

Turtleneck
• 7 •
• 6 •

Cowl
• 7 •
• 6 •

Self-Tie
Ascot
3 • 4 • 7 • 12 (+)
5 • 6 (−)

Open

Wide
(+) 2 • 5 • 6 • 8
(−) 3 • 4 • 7 • 11

Sailor
2 • 6 • 8
3 • 7

Winged • Poet
2 • 6 • 7 • 8
• 3 •

Teardrop
3 • 6
2 • 7 • 11

Closed

Peter Pan
• 7 •
• 6 •

Pointed
• 7 • (+)
• 6 • (−)

Lapels

Notched
(+) 3 • 4 • 6
(−) • 7 •

Peaked
2 • 4 • 6 • 8
3 • 7

Chelsea
3 • 4 • 6
2 • 5 • 7 • 11 • 12

Shawl • Roll • Tuxedo
3 • 4 • 6 (+)
2 • 5 • 7 • 11 • 12 (−)

Tips: Neck accessories, page 83, may turn a minus (−) into a plus (+).

Figure Problem #6: Repeating curved lines near your face will emphasize facial roundness. See page 34.

Figure Problem #7: Turn your collars up! Wear short necklaces.

Refer to these illustrations to evaluate the sleeve styles in:

Blouses
Shirts
Tops
Jackets
Coats
Dresses

Classic Shirt

(+) 9 • 10
(−)

Bishop

3 • 9 • 10
2 • 15 • 18

Bell • Angel

3 • 10
2 • 9 • 18

Raglan

• 3 •
2 • 8 • 11 • 12 • 18

Dolman • Batwing

2 • 9 • 18
3 • 8 • 11

Kimono

2 • 12 • 18   (+)
3 • 8 • 9 • 11   (−)

Puffed • Peasant • Gibson

(+) 2 • 8 • 18
(−) 3 • 9 • 10 • 11

Padded Shoulder

2 • 8 • 10 • 18
• 3 •

Epaulets

2 • 8 • 18
• 3 •

Cuffed • Tabbed

9 • 12
3 • 10 • 11

Cuffs

3 • 9   (+)
2 • 10 • 18   (−)

Tips: Figure Problems #2 and #8. Always use shoulder pads when possible to create a more positive shoulder silhouette.
Figure Problems #9 and #10. Avoid sleeve fabrics that are sheer, stretchy, or clinging.

Sleeve Lengths

A Sleeveless
B Extended
C Short
D ½
E ¾
F Long
G Cuffed

	A	B	C	D	E	F	G
+		2 • 18	12	12	3 • 9 10	3 • 9 10	3 • 9
−	2 • 3 • 8 9 • 10	8 • 9 10	3 • 9 10 • 11	9 • 10	2		2 • 10 18

Sabrina • Halter

(+)
(−) 2 • 3 • 8 • 9
10 • 11 • 12 • 18

Petal

2 • 8 • 18
3 • 10 • 11

Bell

2 • 12 • 18
3 • 9 • 10 • 11

Capped • Butterfly

2 • 18   (+)
3 • 8 • 9 • 10   (−)

These styles focus on tops that show how your torso may be emphasized or hidden.

Evaluate additional styles and variations by referring to:

Necklines
Collars
Lapels
Sleeves
Sleeve Lengths

Timeless Classics

Style lines that flatter most figures stay in style longer than less-flattering lines. This blouse is a flattering combination of:

Notched collar
High yoke with gathers
Long, cuffed sleeves

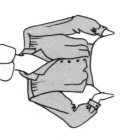

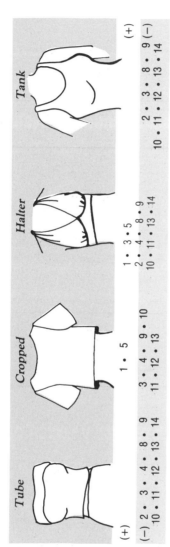

Tube

(+)
(−) 2 • 3 • 4 • 8 • 9
10 • 11 • 12 • 13 • 14

Cropped

1 • 5

3 • 4 • 9 • 10
11 • 12 • 13

Halter

1 • 3 • 5

2 • 4 • 8 • 9
10 • 11 • 13 • 14

Tank

(+)

2 • 3 • 8 • 9 (−)
10 • 11 • 12 • 13 • 14

Emphasizes Bustline and Waist

Basque

(+) 4 • 16
(−) 1 • 2 • 5 • 11
13 • 14 • 15 • 18

Western

4 • 8 • 12

1 • 2 • 3 • 5
11 • 13 • 14 • 15 • 18

Belted Tunic/Shirt

3 • 5 • 12 • 16

1 • 2 • 4 • 13
14 • 15 • 18

Emphasizes Waist and Hips

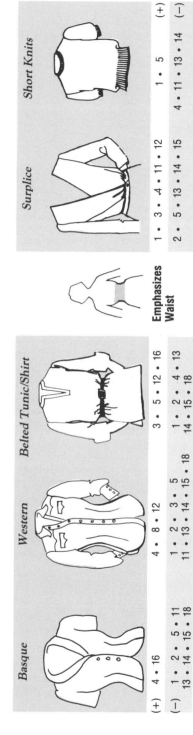

Surplice

1 • 3 • 4 • 11 • 12

2 • 5 • 13 • 14 • 15

Short Knits

4 • 11 • 13 • 14

1 • 5

(+)

(−)

Emphasizes Waist

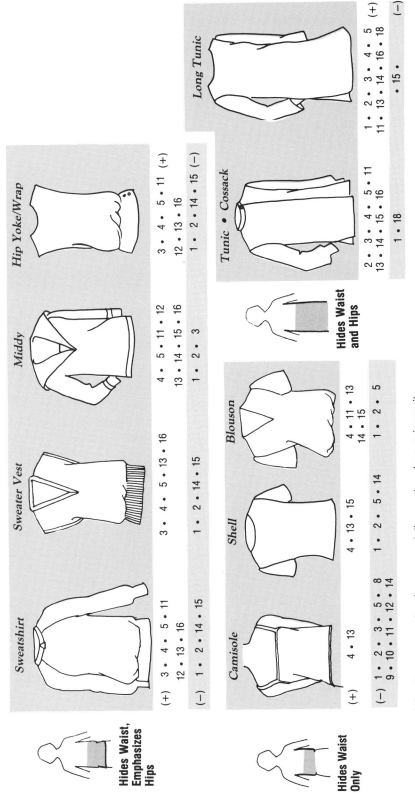

Sweatshirt

(+) 3 • 4 • 5 • 11
12 • 13 • 16

(–) 1 • 2 • 14 • 15

Sweater Vest

3 • 4 • 5 • 13 • 16

1 • 2 • 14 • 15

Middy

4 • 5 • 11 • 12
13 • 14 • 15 • 16

1 • 2 • 3

Hip Yoke/Wrap

3 • 4 • 5 • 11 (+)
12 • 13 • 16

1 • 2 • 14 • 15 (–)

Hides Waist, Emphasizes Hips

Long Tunic

1 • 2 • 3 • 4 • 5 (+)
11 • 13 • 14 • 16 • 18

• 15 • (–)

Tunic • Cossack

2 • 3 • 4 • 5 • 11
13 • 14 • 15 • 16

1 • 18

Hides Waist and Hips

Camisole

(+) 1 • 2 • 3 • 5 • 8
9 • 10 • 11 • 12 • 14

Shell

4 • 13 • 15

1 • 2 • 5 • 14

Blouson

4 • 11 • 13
14 • 15

1 • 2 • 5

Hides Waist Only

When tops are sewn to a lower garment, they create a dress or jumpsuit. As separates, they can be used in combinations with many skirts, pants, and suits to create fabulous outfits. Wearing your plus (+) tops over the tops of skirts and pants that are a minus (–) for you will expand your wardrobe possibilities.

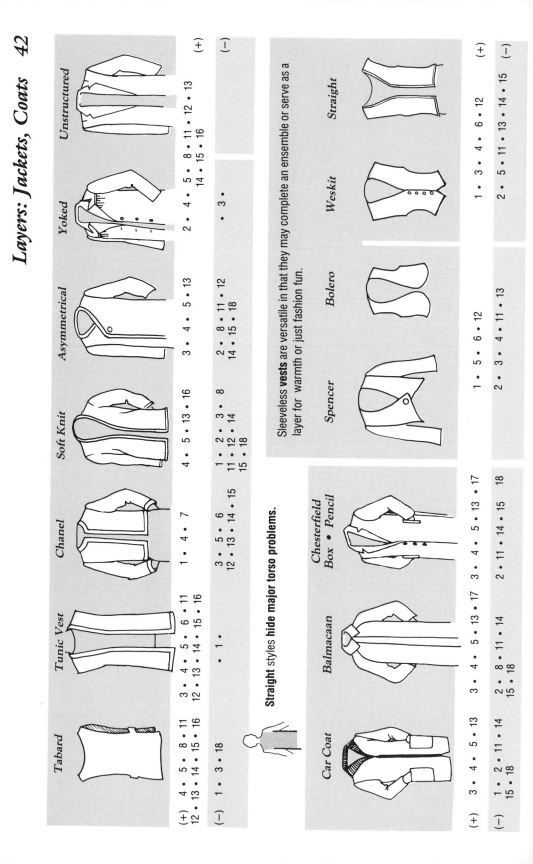

Tabard
(+) 4 • 5 • 8 • 11 • 12 • 13 • 14 • 15 • 16
(−) 1 • 3 • 18

Tunic Vest
(+) 3 • 4 • 5 • 6 • 11 • 12 • 13 • 14 • 15 • 16
(−) • 1 •

Chanel
(+) 1 • 4 • 7
(−) 3 • 5 • 6 • 12 • 13 • 14 • 15

Soft Knit
(+) 4 • 5 • 13 • 16
(−) 1 • 2 • 3 • 8 • 11 • 12 • 14 • 15 • 18

Asymmetrical
(+) 3 • 4 • 5 • 13
(−) 2 • 8 • 11 • 12 • 14 • 15 • 18

Yoked
(+) 2 • 4 • 5 • 8 • 11 • 12 • 13 • 14 • 15 • 16
(−) • 3 •

Unstructured
(+)
(−)

Straight styles **hide major torso problems.**

Car Coat
(+) 3 • 4 • 5 • 13
(−) 1 • 2 • 11 • 14 • 15 • 18

Balmacaan
(+) 3 • 4 • 5 • 13 • 17
(−) 2 • 8 • 11 • 14 • 15 • 18

Chesterfield • Box • Pencil
(+) 3 • 4 • 5 • 13 • 17
(−) 2 • 11 • 14 • 15 • 18

Sleeveless **vests** are versatile in that they may complete an ensemble or serve as a layer for warmth or just fashion fun.

Spencer
(+) 1 • 5 • 6 • 12
(−) 2 • 3 • 4 • 11 • 13

Bolero

Weskit
(+) 1 • 3 • 4 • 6 • 12
(−) 2 • 5 • 11 • 13 • 14 • 15

Straight
(+)
(−)

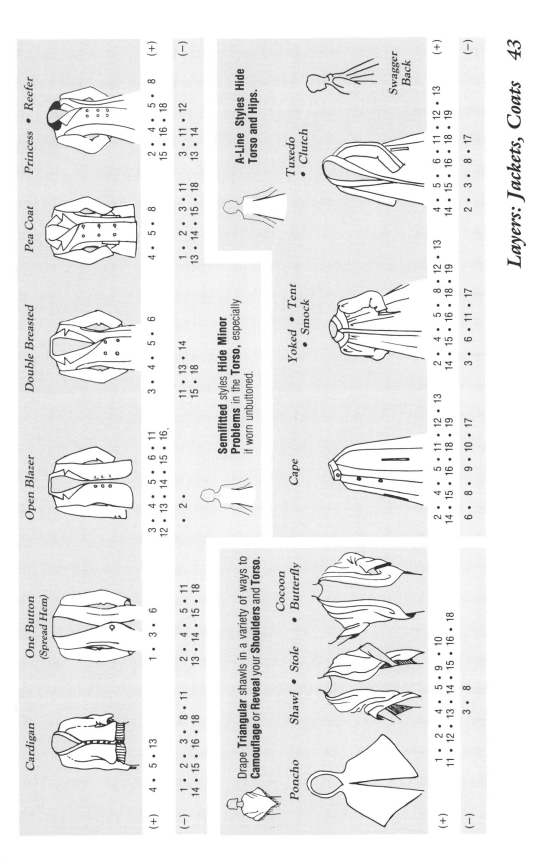

Top row styles:

Cardigan • *One Button* (Spread Hem) • *Open Blazer* • *Double Breasted* • *Pea Coat* • *Princess* • *Reefer*

Cardigan
(+) 4 • 5 • 13
(−) 1 • 2 • 3 • 8 • 11 • 14 • 15 • 16 • 18

One Button (Spread Hem)
(+) 1 • 3 • 6
(−) 2 • 4 • 5 • 11 • 13 • 14 • 15 • 18

Open Blazer
(+) 3 • 4 • 5 • 6 • 11 • 12 • 13 • 14 • 15 • 16.
(−) • 2

Double Breasted
(+) 3 • 4 • 5 • 6
(−) 11 • 13 • 14 • 15 • 18

Pea Coat
(+) 4 • 5 • 8
(−) 1 • 2 • 3 • 14 • 13 • 14 • 15 • 18

Princess • Reefer
(+) 2 • 4 • 5 • 8 • 15 • 16 • 18
(−) 3 • 11 • 12 • 13 • 14

Semifitted styles **Hide Minor Problems** in the **Torso**, especially if worn unbuttoned.

Drape **Triangular** shawls in a variety of ways to **Camouflage** or **Reveal** your **Shoulders** and **Torso**.

Poncho • *Shawl* • *Stole* • *Cocoon* • *Butterfly*

Poncho
(+) 1 • 2 • 4 • 5 • 9 • 10 • 11 • 12 • 13 • 14 • 15 • 16 • 18
(−) 3 • 8

Shawl • Stole • Cocoon • Butterfly
(+) 1 • 2 • 3 • 4 • 5 • 11 • 12 • 13 • 14 • 15 • 16 • 18
(−) 3 • 8

A-Line Styles Hide Torso and Hips.

Tuxedo • Clutch • *Yoked • Tent • Smock* • *Cape* • *Swagger Back*

Cape
(+) 2 • 4 • 5 • 11 • 12 • 13 • 14 • 15 • 16 • 18 • 19
(−) 6 • 8 • 9 • 10 • 17

Yoked • Tent • Smock
(+) 2 • 4 • 5 • 8 • 12 • 13 • 14 • 15 • 16 • 18 • 19
(−) 3 • 6 • 11 • 17

Tuxedo • Clutch
(+) 4 • 5 • 6 • 11 • 12 • 13 • 14 • 15 • 16 • 18 • 19
(−) 2 • 3 • 8 • 17

Layers: Jackets, Coats 44

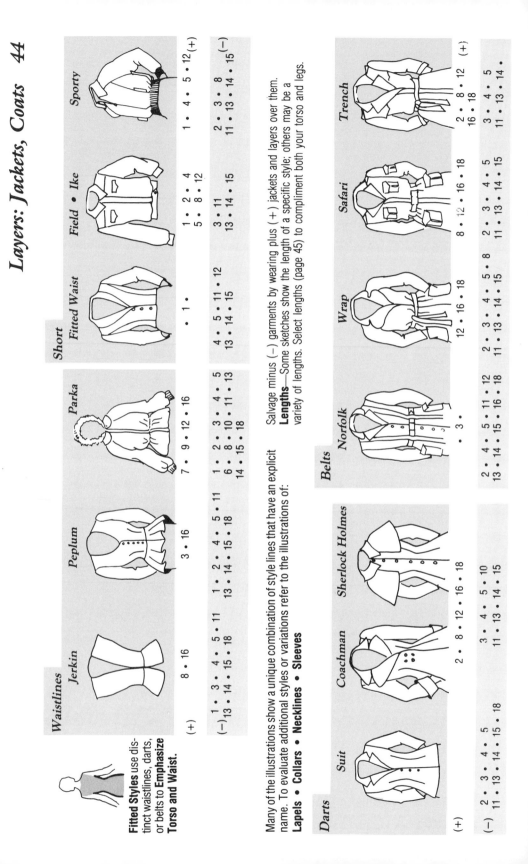

Fitted Styles use distinct waistlines, darts, or belts to **Emphasize Torso and Waist.**

Waistlines

Jerkin

(+) 8 · 16

(−) 1 · 3 · 4 · 5 · 11
    13 · 14 · 15 · 18

Peplum

3 · 16

1 · 2 · 4 · 5 · 11
13 · 14 · 15 · 18

Parka

7 · 9 · 12 · 16

1 · 2 · 3 · 4 · 5
6 · 8 · 10 · 11 · 13
14 · 15 · 18

Short

Fitted Waist

· 1 ·

4 · 5 · 11 · 12
13 · 14 · 15

Field · Ike

1 · 2 · 4
5 · 8 · 12

3 · 11
13 · 14 · 15

Sporty

1 · 4 · 5 · 12 (+)

2 · 3 · 8
11 · 13 · 14 · 15 (−)

Many of the illustrations show a unique combination of style lines that have an explicit name. To evaluate additional styles or variations refer to the illustrations of:
Lapels · Collars · Necklines · Sleeves

Salvage minus (−) garments by wearing plus (+) jackets and layers over them.
Lengths—Some sketches show the length of a specific style; others may be a variety of lengths. Select lengths (page 45) to compliment both your torso and legs.

Darts

Suit

(+) 2 · 3 · 4 · 5

(−) 11 · 13 · 14 · 15 · 18

Coachman

3 · 4 · 5

11 · 13 · 14 · 15

Sherlock Holmes

2 · 8 · 12 · 16 · 18

3 · 4 · 5 · 10
11 · 13 · 14 · 15

Belts

Norfolk

· 3 ·

2 · 4 · 5 · 11 · 12
13 · 14 · 15 · 16 · 18

Wrap

12 · 16 · 18

2 · 3 · 4 · 5 · 14 · 15
11 · 13 · 14 · 15

Safari

8 · 12 · 16 · 18

2 · 3 · 4 · 5
11 · 13 · 14 · 15

Trench

2 · 8 · 12 (+)
16 · 18

3 · 4 · 5
11 · 13 · 14 ·

The length of your top garment will determine how long your upper torso, lower torso, and legs look. To create interesting suit combinations, wear short jackets with longer skirts—and long jackets with shorter skirts. To minimize the impact of a horizontal hemline on the broadest part of your hips, combine tops and bottoms that are the same or similar colors.

Lengths: Tops, Jackets, Coats

	Cropped	Waist	Hipbone	Midhip	Below the Hip	3/4	7/8	Midcalf	Long	Evening Maxi
(+)		1 • 2 • 5	1 • 2 • 4	3 • 4 • 16	2 • 13 • 14	2 • 13 • 14 18	1 • 2 • 13 14 • 15 • 18	17	1 • 17 19	1 • 17 (+) 19
(−)	3 • 4 • 11 • 13		5 • 13	1 • 2 • 18	1 • 18	1		19		(−)

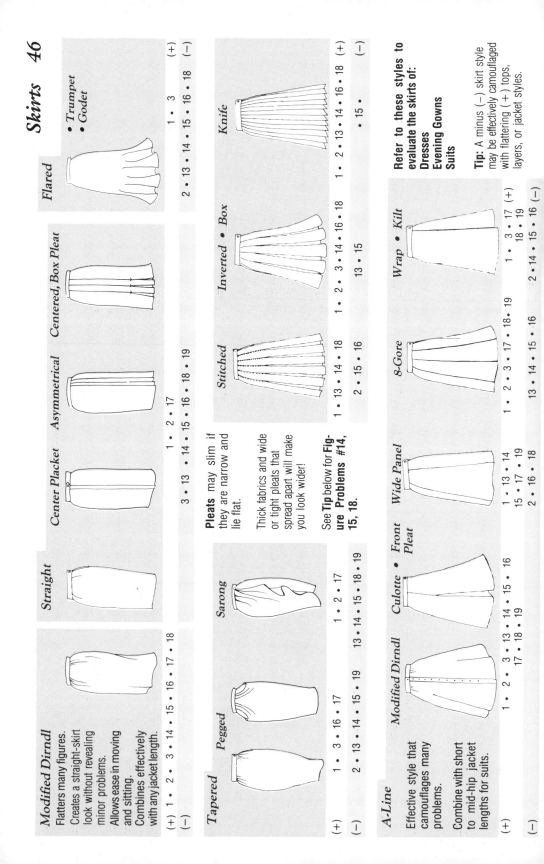

Modified Dirndl

Flatters many figures.

Creates a straight-skirt look without revealing minor problems.

Allows ease in moving and sitting.

Combines effectively with any jacket length.

(+) 1 • 2 • 3 • 14 • 15 • 16 • 17 • 18
(−)

Straight

Center Placket   Asymmetrical   Centered, Box Pleat

(+)   1 • 2 • 17
(−) 3 • 13 • 14 • 15 • 16 • 18 • 19

Flared

• Trumpet
• Godet

(+) 1 • 3
(−) 2 • 13 • 14 • 15 • 16 • 18

Tapered

Pegged   Sarong

(+) 1 • 3 • 16 • 17   1 • 2 • 17
(−) 2 • 13 • 14 • 15 • 19   13 • 14 • 15 • 18 • 19

Pleats may slim if they are narrow and lie flat.

Thick fabrics and wide or tight pleats that spread apart will make you look wider!

See **Tip** below for **Figure Problems #14, 15, 18.**

Stitched   Inverted • Box

(+) 1 • 13 • 14 • 18   1 • 2 • 3 • 14 • 16 • 18
(−) 2 • 15 • 16   13 • 15

Knife

(+) 1 • 2 • 13 • 14 • 16 • 18
(−) • 15

A-Line

Effective style that camouflages many problems.

Combine with short to mid-hip jacket lengths for suits.

Modified Dirndl   Culotte • Front Pleat   Wide Panel

(+) 1 • 2 • 3 • 13 • 14 • 15 • 16   1 • 13 • 14 • 15 • 16   1 • 13 • 14 • 15 • 17 • 19
    17 • 18 • 19   17 • 18 • 19
(−) 2 • 16 • 18

8-Gore   Wrap • Kilt

(+) 1 • 2 • 3 • 17 • 18 • 19   1 • 3 • 17 • 18 • 19
(−) 13 • 14 • 15 • 16   2 • 13 • 14 • 15 • 16

Refer to these styles to evaluate the skirts of:
Dresses
Evening Gowns
Suits

Tip: A minus (−) skirt style may be effectively camouflaged with flattering (+) tops, layers, or jacket styles.

Full

	Dirndl-Gathered	Tiered	Flounced	Circular	Yoked • Drop Waist
(+)	3 • 15 • 16 • 18	3 • 13 • 15 • 16 • 18	2 • 3 • 13 • 15 • 16 • 18		3 • 4
(−)	2 • 13 • 14	1 • 2 • 14 • 17 • 19	14 • 17		1 • 2 • 5 • 13 • 16 / 14 • 15 • 16

TIP: Figure Problem #1. To avoid looking "legless," show more ankle when wearing a waltz length or long skirt. Wear a medium or high heel with longer lengths of skirts.

	Costume	Mini	Above the Knee	Below the Knee	Midcalf	Tea Waltz		Evening
Skirt	Costume	Mini	Bermuda Walking	Pedal Pushers Clam Diggers	Toreador	Cropped	Cuffed	Long
Pants	Shorts Jamaican			Capri				

	Costume	Mini	Above the Knee	Below the Knee	Midcalf	Tea Waltz	Cuffed	Evening
(+)	1		1 • 17 / 18 • 19	1 • 17 / 19		17	17	1 • 17 • 19
(−)	2 • 5 • 14 • 15 / 17 • 18 • 19	1 • 2 • 5 / 15 • 17 / 18 • 19		19	19		1 • 19	

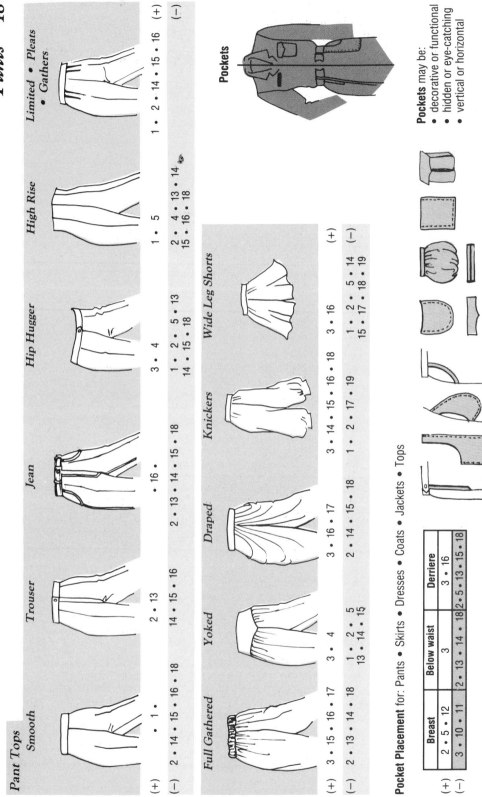

Pant Tops

Smooth — **Trouser** — **Jean** — **Hip Hugger** — **High Rise** — **Limited • Pleats • Gathers**

	Smooth	Trouser	Jean	Hip Hugger	High Rise	Limited • Pleats • Gathers
(+)	• 1 •	2 • 13	• 16 •	3 • 4	1 • 5	1 • 2 • 14 • 15 • 16
(–)	2 • 14 • 15 • 16 • 18	14 • 15 • 16	2 • 13 • 14 • 15 • 18	1 • 2 • 5 • 13 / 14 • 15 • 18	2 • 4 • 13 • 14 / 15 • 16 • 18	

Full Gathered — **Yoked** — **Draped** — **Knickers** — **Wide Leg Shorts**

	Full Gathered	Yoked	Draped	Knickers	Wide Leg Shorts
(+)	3 • 15 • 16 • 17	3 • 4	3 • 16 • 17	3 • 14 • 15 • 16 • 18	3 • 16
(–)	2 • 13 • 14 • 18	1 • 2 • 5 / 13 • 14 • 15	2 • 14 • 15 • 18	1 • 2 • 17 • 19	1 • 2 • 5 • 14 / 15 • 17 • 18 • 19

Pockets

Pockets may be:
- decorative or functional
- hidden or eye-catching
- vertical or horizontal

Pocket Placement for: Pants • Skirts • Dresses • Coats • Jackets • Tops

	Breast	Below waist	Derriere
(+)	2 • 5 • 12	3	3 • 16
(–)	3 • 10 • 11	2 • 13 • 14 • 18	2 • 5 • 13 • 15 • 18

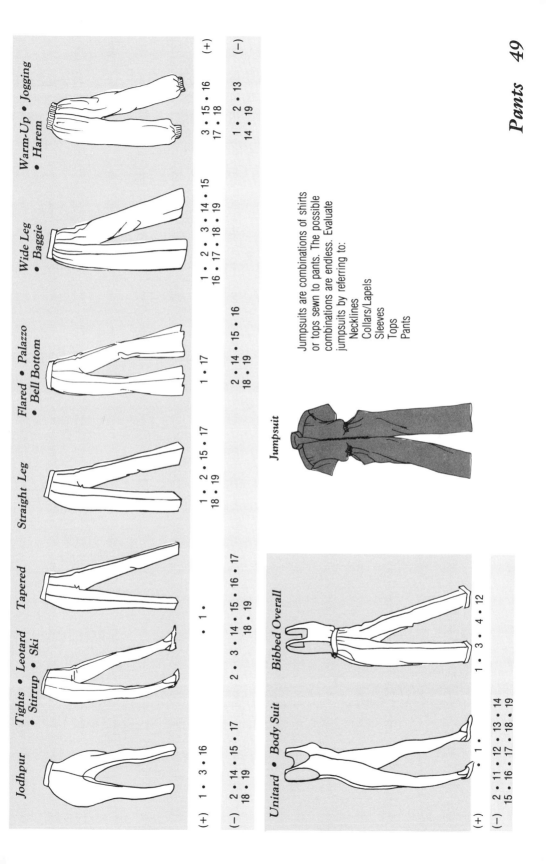

Pants   49

Jodhpur

(+) 1 • 3 • 16

(−) 2 • 14 • 15 • 17
18 • 19

Tights • Leotard • Stirrup • Ski

(+) • 1 •

(−) 2 • 3 • 14 • 15 • 16 • 17
18 • 19

Tapered

(+) • 1 •

(−) 2 • 3 • 14 • 15 • 16 • 17
18 • 19

Straight Leg

(+) 1 • 2 • 15 • 17
18 • 19

Flared • Palazzo • Bell Bottom

(+) 1 • 17

(−) 2 • 14 • 15 • 16
18 • 19

Wide Leg • Baggie

(+) 1 • 2 • 3 • 14 • 15
16 • 17 • 18 • 19

Warm-Up • Jogging • Harem

(+) 3 • 15 • 16
17 • 18

(−) 1 • 2 • 13
14 • 19

Unitard • Body Suit

(+) • 1 •

(−) 2 • 11 • 12 • 13 • 14
15 • 16 • 17 • 18 • 19

Bibbed Overall

(+) 1 • 3 • 4 • 12

(−) 1 • 3 • 16

Jumpsuit

Jumpsuits are combinations of shirts or tops sewn to pants. The possible combinations are endless. Evaluate jumpsuits by referring to:
  Necklines
  Collars/Lapels
  Sleeves
  Tops
  Pants

Descending Waistlines

	Sundress	Empire	Peasant	Jumper	Blouson	Fitted Dropped Waist	Tabard	Chemise
(+)	1 • 5 • 16	1 • 2 • 4 • 5 • 13 • 18 / 14 • 15 • 16	5 • 12	3 • 4 / 8 • 12	4 • 11 • 12 • 13 / 14 • 15 • 16	3 • 4 • 5 • 11 / 12 • 13 • 16	3 • 4 • 5 / 12 • 13	3 • 4 • 5 / 11 • 13 • 16
(−)	2 • 3 • 8 • 9 / 10 • 11 • 12 • 13 / 14 • 15 • 18	3 • 10 • 11 / 14 • 15 • 16 • 18	3 • 4 • 11 / 13 • 14	2 • 5 / 11 • 13	1 • 5	1 • 2 • 14 • 15	1 • 2 • 14 / 15 • 16	1 • 2 • 12 • 14 / 15 • 18 • 19 / **Read Tip**

No Waistlines

	Unbelted Shift	Float	Yoked • Caftan • Tent • Mu-Mu
(+)	1 • 4 • 5 / 11 • 13 • 16	1 • 2 • 3 • 4 • 5 / 11 • 12 • 13 • 14 / 15 • 16 • 18 • 19	1 • 4 • 5 • 12 / 13 • 14 • 15 • 16 / 18 • 19
(−)	2 • 12 / 14 • 15 • 18 / **Read Tip**	17	2 • 3 • 11 • 17

Suggested Waistlines

	Fitted Sheath • Princess	A-Line • Princess	Coatdress • Surplice • Wrap
(+)	1 • 4	1 • 2 • 4 • 5 / 15 • 16 • 18	1 • 3 • 4 / 5 • 13 • 16
(−)	2 • 3 • 5 / 11 • 12 • 13 • 14 / 15 • 16 • 18	11 • 12 / 13 • 14	2 • 11 • 12 / 14 • 15

When tops and skirts are sewn together they become a dress or an evening gown. These show basic torso silhouettes that may be available in a variety of details.

To evaluate additional dress details refer to:
Tops, Necklines, Sleeves, Collars, Belts, Skirts/Lengths

TIP: Straight dresses should fit with ease. Tight garments will reveal figure problems.

Patterns can help or reveal your torso problems:

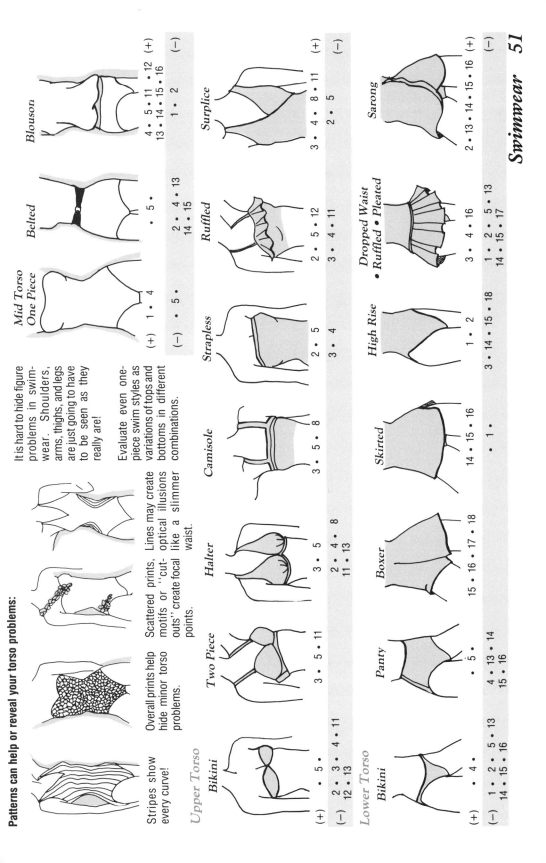

Stripes show every curve!

Overall prints help hide minor torso problems.

Scattered prints, motifs or "cut-outs" create focal points.

Lines may create optical illusions like a slimmer waist.

It is hard to hide figure problems in swim-wear. Shoulders, arms, thighs, and legs are just going to have to be seen as they really are!

Evaluate even one-piece swim styles as variations of tops and bottoms in different combinations.

Upper Torso

Bikini
(+) • 5 •
(−) • 2 • 3 • 4 • 11
      12 • 13

Two Piece
3 • 5 • 11

Halter
3 • 5
2 • 4 • 8
11 • 13

Camisole
3 • 5 • 8
3 • 4

Strapless
2 • 5
3 • 4

Ruffled
2 • 5 • 12
3 • 4 • 11

Surplice
(+) 3 • 4 • 8 • 11
(−) 2 • 5

Mid Torso One Piece
(+) 1 • 4
(−) • 5 •

Belted
• 5 •
2 • 4 • 13
14 • 15

Blouson
(+) 4 • 5 • 11 • 12
    13 • 14 • 15 • 16
(−) 1 • 2

Lower Torso

Bikini
(+) • 4 •
(−) 1 • 2 • 5 • 13
    14 • 15 • 16

Panty
• 5 •
4 • 13 • 14
15 • 16

Boxer
15 • 16 • 17 • 18

Skirted
14 • 15 • 16
• 1 •

High Rise
1 • 2
3 • 14 • 15 • 18

Dropped Waist • Ruffled • Pleated
3 • 4 • 16
1 • 2 • 5 • 13
14 • 15 • 17

Sarong
(+) 2 • 13 • 14 • 15 • 16
(−)

THE KEY TO THE STYLES THAT FLATTER YOUR FIGURE

What do all those (+)'s and (−)'s mean?

The styles you have just marked have been analyzed according to their potential to flatter your own unique combination of figure problems.

A summary of this key is located on the cover foldout flap.

(+) = Flattering Styles
( ) = Acceptable Styles
(−) = Detracting Styles

(+) The Plus Row: Flattering Styles That *Add* to Your Appearance

If you have circled one or more of your figure problem numbers in the plus (+) row, it means that the style (as illustrated) will visually *correct or camouflage the figure problems* circled under it. It flatters your figure. *Buy, sew, or order these styles.*

( ) The Neutral Zone: Acceptable Styles

If your figure problem numbers are *not listed* under a specific style, it means that *the illustrated style neither corrects nor emphasizes that figure problem.* For example, Figure Problem #1 is not listed under any neckline styles, as there are no necklines that will make your legs look longer! Unlisted numbers ( ) represent "neutral" styles that may actually be very flattering. *Try them!*

(−) The Minus Row: Detracting Styles That *Subtract* from Your Appearance

The lines of these styles *reveal or emphasize the figure problems* listed under them. They "take away" from your potential. These styles create a visual challenge. When you wear them, you will have to work harder to look good! To salvage Detracting Styles, try combining or layering the minus (−) styles with plus (+) styles that are more eye-catching. **You should avoid a minus (−) style *only* if the minus (−) remains obvious and continues to detract from your appearance.**

Example: Turn to pages 40–41, which shows a selection of tops. See how many figure problem numbers are listed in the (−) row under the camisole (camisoles reveal more than they conceal). Even if you have several figure problems circled under the camisole, **a (−) does not mean you should not buy or wear it. It just indicates that *you should not wear it by itself.*** Wear the camisole under a flattering jacket. Just don't take the jacket off!

A variety of solutions on how to correct, camouflage, and salvage the
(−) parts of your wardrobe are explored in Chapter 4.

(+) and (−) Styles That Conflict: They Are Both Flattering
and Detracting on You

Because most women have three to seven figure problems to consider
in selecting clothing, it is often difficult to find a garment that camouflages *every* figure challenge. The more figure problems you have, the
more likely it is that you will have styles that are a (+) *for some figure
problems and a (−) for other ones.* This means that only a part of you will
look good in that style while another part will look worse!

You will be learning how to combine (+) and (−) styles to flatter
your entire figure in the next chapter.

WILL A FASHION TREND BECOME A FIASCO OR A FAVORITE?

Look through the pages in the Style Guide each shopping season to
discover how the latest fashions will look on you.

High-fashion trends tend to focus on a specific part of the body such
as shoulders or legs and may distort body proportions on purpose. Just
because a style is "in vogue" does not mean that everyone looks
fantastic in it. If the style lines are negative for a woman's figure, a chic
garment may make her look ridiculous rather than fashionable.

Trends that flatter many figure problems usually stay in vogue longer
than those that flatter few figures. (Padded shoulders are an example.)
Check how many of the nineteen figure problem numbers are listed in
the (+) row under a "fashion forward" style to determine if it will stay
in vogue long enough to warrant a major expenditure. If it is a (+)
style for many problems *and it flatters you,* the sooner you buy it, the
more "wearings per dollar" you will have before it passes from the
fashion scene.

OTHER WAYS TO FIGURE OUT FASHIONS

The Style Evaluation Chart: Evaluating Additional Garments

Although there are more than 230 specific style illustrations in the
Style Guide, it would be impossible to include every variation of every
style. Many dresses, for example, are combinations of the top and skirt
illustrations. You can evaluate additional garments that are not illustrated in the Style Guide by using the Style Evaluation Chart at the end
of this chapter.

A quick reference guide to the most flattering style lines for your figure can be found inside the back cover. Follow the directions on page 98, and complete the "Style Lines That Flatter My Figure" section of your Figure Chart. Then compare the lines drawn on the figure to the most obvious lines of a garment. You will be able to see instantly if the lines are compatible with your figure.

The Blink Test: How to See Style Lines and Designs Instantly

The Blink Test is an easy way to see the most eye-catching line and design elements of a garment in only three seconds.

1. Hang the garment 5 feet away from you.
2. Close your eyes and count to three (a long blink). Open them.
3. *Instantly* what do you see first?

Your eyes will automatically go toward the most noticeable part of the garment: The Focal Point. Focal Points may be created by style lines, shapes, prints, colors, or even texture.

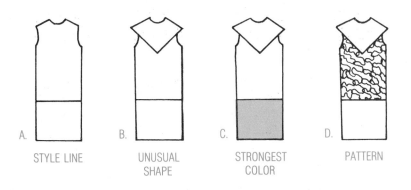

A. STYLE LINE B. UNUSUAL SHAPE C. STRONGEST COLOR D. PATTERN

Notice how the style line in A loses your attention as a more eye-catching collar is combined with it in B (hello, face). In C the collar loses your attention due to a color change (hello, legs). In D the eye goes to the busy pattern in the center of the dress (hello, torso).

You will be learning more about how to use the Blink Test and focal points to accent your assets in the chapters that follow.

A WORKBOOK THAT WORKS FOR YOU

You now have four ways to figure out fashions and how they relate to your figure:
For specific styles and details use:

- The Style Guide, pages 35–51.
- The Style Evaluation Chart at the end of this chapter.

For quick reference use:

- The Figure Chart, page 99.
- The Blink Test, pages 89–90.

Use any or all of them to shop, order, or sew your wardrobe.

SHOPPING. To avoid "dressing room despair," tuck your workbook in your handbag and evaluate garments *before* you go to the dressing room. Ask the sales staff to help you find garments that have similar style lines to the lines drawn on your Figure Chart on page 99.

ORDERING. Remove the fear of ordering the wrong thing from a mail-order catalog or television retailing channel. Follow the company's size charts, then order with confidence. What a pleasure it will be to open the box, slip the garments on, and smile—because you ordered "keepers!"

SEWING. "Is there anyone out there with an unfinished sewing disaster tucked in a drawer?" When I asked this question of more than 400 home economics teachers at their national convention, I was amazed when almost every one of those textile professionals raised their hands. Even experts who teach garment construction have discovered that a perfectly fitted garment made with the most fabulous fabric is a sewing mistake when the pattern they selected is unflattering on them. *Flatter Your Figure* takes the guesswork out of picking a pattern. It saves time, money, effort, and disappointment. *FYF* also gives dressmakers the wonderful advantage of knowing which patterns to combine to create an outfit that flatters the entire figure. No more sewing mistakes!

Now that you know how to figure out fashions, on to Chapter 4 to discover how to use illusions to create a little figure magic on your figure—today!

STYLE EVALUATION CHART

Use this chart to evaluate garments not illustrated in the Style Guide. It is especially helpful in choosing mail-order items and patterns.

1. Turn to the Style Guide page indicated below and find the illustration that most closely resembles each *part* of the garment.
2. If you have a figure problem circled under it, look at the list of figure problems on the cover flap to see what part of the body that number refers to.
   a. Draw a "(+)" on top of the figures below where the style is FLATTERING (+) for your figure.
   b. Draw a "(−)" on top of the figures below where the style is DETRACTING (−) for your figure.
      Now you can easily see where the style will be a plus or a minus on you.
3. Garments that flatter every part of your figure are rare. Most clothing requires some additions or changes to become totally flattering. Note under IMPROVEMENT any garments or accessories you need to correct, camouflage, or divert attention from any detracting (−) part of the style.

Style	Page	+ or − Tip: Use Pencil	Improvement (add or change)
Neckline	37, 38		
Sleeves	39		
Top/Layer	40, 41		
Jacket/Coat	42–44		
Length	45		
Dress	50		
Skirt	46–47		
Pant	48, 49		
Length	47		
Pockets	48		
Belt	82		
Fabric	67–68		
Pattern	51, 68–69		
Color	54, 70, 76		

Do the Blink Test (pages 89–90). Are the (−)s easy to correct or camouflage? If so: buy, order, or sew it. If the (−)s remain obvious, the garment or ensemble will not be your best investment.

CHAPTER
4

Flattering Your Figure—Today

GETTING DRESSED

"What should I wear?" Dressing decisions confront every woman every day. Getting dressed isn't the problem. The challenge is to get dressed, look in the mirror, and smile at the results.

What keeps women from getting dressed and loving the results?

I have discovered that you don't have to have a crooked back, as I did, to develop a negative attitude toward your body. I have met hundreds of women, some with fantastic figures, who hate their bodies.

On a trip to New York, I met a very overweight young woman. As we discussed our respective businesses she shared her problems with me.

"I hate my body. Two years ago I was an aerobics instructor." Looking at her, I was frankly astonished. She continued, "I was severely injured in a car accident and spent ten months in the hospital. By the time I got out, I had gained 90 pounds. Unfortunately my injuries will keep me from ever exercising again. I hate being fat. But what I hate even more than being heavy now is the fact that I wasted all those years hating my thin, fit body."

The moral to this story: Love your body *now*. It is the best one you have today!

NO BODY'S PERFECT

I used to put myself down constantly about my weight and body condition, especially when I was 4-F. When I started my fashion make-over I decided to take control of my figure, too. Now, the idea of eating less and exercising more is the opposite of what I am inclined to do, but with the help of others, I now have a much better body and habits. The struggle to keep from regaining the 30 pounds I lost is hard, but I've learned not to berate myself when I don't follow my diet and exercise programs perfectly each day. After years of self-abuse, the feeling of self-respect I experience when I choose to do what is good for my body is one I like to repeat. Positive reinforcement, rather than destructive criticism, works when it comes from within as well as from others. Try it. No more put-downs! Treat yourself to a better body— instead of high-calorie treats.

Unlike so many parts of our lives that involve other people, your body and how you dress it are under your absolute control. While you may not have the body you would have ordered if you had a choice, you are the one who chooses each day: what you eat, whether you exercise, what you wear, and how the body you do have will look. Take control of your appearance—because that is just what it is—yours.

DON'T WAIT ON YOUR WEIGHT

Extra pounds are one of the main reasons why millions of women feel frustrated about getting dressed and loving the results. If 5, 25, or 90 pounds are making you feel miserable about your body, you are not alone. Between the ages of twenty and forty-five the average woman gains 19 pounds. Weight gain then slows to about ½ pound per year until age sixty-five, at which time you may actually lose a pound or two (*Statistical Abstract of the United States Government*, 1987).

A clothing chain for large sizes reports that "approximately 47% of American women wear a size 14 or larger." Dr. Richard Landis states in the *American Journal of Clinical Nutrition* (1988) that more than 17 *million* American women are considered obese, which is defined as being 20 percent above ideal weight. Sadly, we are heavier than our mother's generation and our children will be heavier than we are.

Eighty percent of obese children remain obese as adults according to research at the University of California. The focus of the 1990s on healthier bodies should not only be for ourselves but also for our children.

Too many women with weight problems have the attitude that they cannot look good, so why try.

While waiting at a red light one day, I enjoyed watching a fabulous-looking woman cross the street. She probably weighed close to 250 pounds and had very large hips. Her daily choices are to be large and lovely—or large and not so lovely. This woman looked terrific. Her bright red suit and heels were topped off with a big red hat complete with feathers. Her stride and body language said, "I'm happy and confident." Now that was a woman I would like to know.

Staying thin throughout a lifetime is a goal that does elude many of us. That's why learning to cope with the changes in our figures is as much a mental task as a physical one. If some extra pounds do sneak on through the years, focus on maximizing your potential—not your size! Follow the example of the woman above and shun shapeless tents, sacks, and drab colors. Put some pizzazz in your dressing by using the tips in this chapter on prints, color, fit, fabrics, and accessories while tackling those extra pounds. But don't wait until you have reached your goal weight to start looking your best. You can do that today!

CHOICES

There are some aspects of your body you can control—and some you cannot. The wise woman recognizes the difference.

Q. What can you control?

A. Your weight and physical fitness.
If your body condition isn't what you would like it to be, don't get depressed; get the phone book. Assistance from nutrition, exercise, and medical professionals is only a call away. Don't procrastinate another day—both your physical health and self-esteem may be at risk.

Q. What aspects of our bodies are beyond our control?

A. Your height and bone structure.
Genes do show. Don't waste energy fretting over what you cannot change, like the length of your legs or the genetic code that tells each of those extra calories to go directly to your ———. Chances are, the older you get, the more your figure will resemble a relative's.

Have you looked in your mirror lately and seen your mother's body?

The body you saw in your mirror this morning is the one that has to get dressed. By the time you finish this chapter you will know how to dress to:

- Camouflage your figure problems
- Divert attention from problems you cannot camouflage

You will love the results when you know how to get everyone to focus on your assets and ignore your negatives.

CREATING ILLUSIONS WITH CLOTHING

Let's start by tackling the dressing problems associated with extra pounds.

Dressing Thinner

The results of a few extra pounds are

An extra 5 pounds = one dress size larger
An extra 10 pounds = 1 inch thicker body
     . . . especially in certain spots!

It is easy to camouflage about 20 extra pounds with clothing. More than that, the extra weight starts to show in the face and hands. While garments alone cannot make you look 40 pounds lighter, every woman, regardless of her weight, can create the illusion of looking thinner as you can see on the following page.

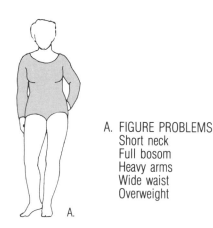

A. FIGURE PROBLEMS
Short neck
Full bosom
Heavy arms
Wide waist
Overweight

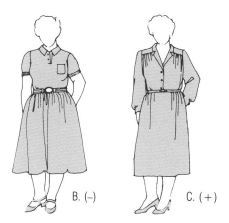
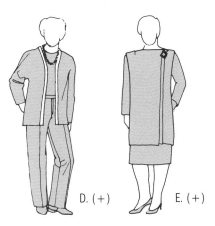

B. (–)   C. (+)   D. (+)   E. (+)

B. DETRACTING

High collar shortens neck
Tight top with breast pocket and short sleeves
Belt that accents her waist
Full dirndl skirt adds volume to her hips
Shoes with straps shorten her legs

Abbra-ca-dab-bra . . .
a slimmer
figure!

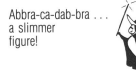

This woman needs to create the illusion of a thinner body. Trace over all the figure-flattering vertical lines created by her clothing in C, D, and E.

For those of you who have extra calorie "hot spots" on the tummy and tush, try these tips:

Tip: Figure Problems #2, 14, 15, and 18

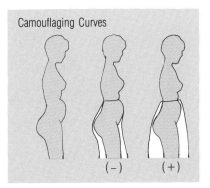

Camouflaging Curves

(–)   (+)

Wear loose skirts that "straighten" unwanted curves rather than cupping around and revealing them. Avoid bias-cut fabrics or spreading pleats that make you look like *you* are spreading! Fit your hips and tummy, not your waist. Loose waistbands are much less noticeable than tight garments.

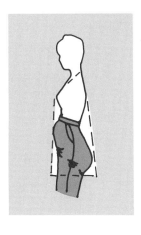

Long, loose, unstructured tops and jackets that *hang straight from the shoulders* can hide many problems.

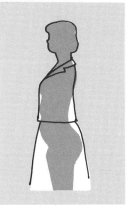

Or, try a short jacket with an A-line skirt.

Even if you have heavy shoulders or arms, add a thin shoulder pad to create the illusion of a corner rather than a curve. (Hint: the blunt end is placed at the shoulder edge.)

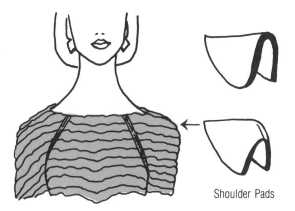

Shoulder Pads

Wear blunt-edge pads under crisp or suit-weight fabrics.

Wear soft-edge pads under knit or draping fabrics.

Pads = Posture improvement for **Figure Problem #8.**

DRESSING A THINNER FIGURE

When I was testing the stick-and-string method on a group of women at a spa, I noticed that figure problems do not discriminate. Even women who are fit and slim can have proportional problems, as the figure below shows.

A. FIGURE PROBLEMS
Short legs for body
Wide shoulders
Long neck (short hairstyle
    elongates neck)
Long waist

B and C. The torso is shortened
or narrowed with collars, bows,
belts, pockets, and seam lines.
The legs are elongated by wearing
slender skirts and vertical pleats.

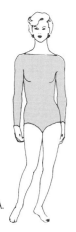
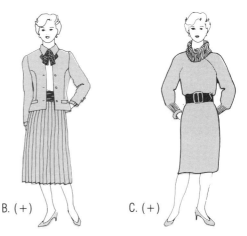

A.   B. (+)   C. (+)

D. DETRACTING STYLES
Scooped neck
Puffed sleeves
Vertical lines on top
Low belt and hemline
Cropped pants
High-vamp shoes

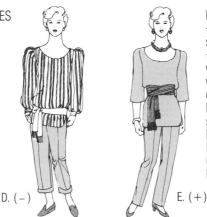

E. CORRECTIONS
★ Add a short necklace to
shorten her neck.
★ Shorten the torso by
wearing the belt at the
waistline. Break up the low
detracting (–) horizontal
hemline by letting the tas-
sels extend over it. Note
how much longer her legs
look.
Cuffless long pants
Low-vamp shoes

D. (–)   E. (+)

★ CONCEPT shown in E: A detracting (–) style is easily camouflaged when the flattering (+) style combined with it is more obvious.

DRESSING TO BALANCE YOUR PROPORTIONS

One woman I met at the spa when I was doing the research for *FYF* is a good example of how to dress a body whose upper and lower torso are not in proportion. Elaine's trim figure will always have broad hips. No amount of weight loss or exercise will make her pelvic bones move closer together. What she *can* control is choosing clothing that creates the illusion of balanced hips and shoulders, like the woman below.

Many women require opposing style lines to widen and lengthen different parts of the body. Observe how this woman uses line, shape, and volume to enlarge her smaller upper torso while visually slimming or diverting attention away from her wider hips.

Style lines needed to create the illusion of:

Wider shoulders
Fuller bust
Longer waist
Slimmer hips and thighs

Note: The lines drawn on this figure are an example of how to draw the lines on your Figure Chart section titled "Style Lines That Flatter My Figure," in the back of the book on page 99.

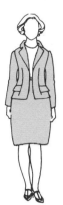 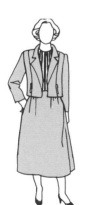 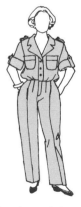

A. Pitiful

B. Figure flattering head to toe

C. Blouson top with horizontal design; A-line skirt with verticals on bottom

D. Lapels, pockets, cuffs, and tabs create volume and width on top. Buttons, placket, and pant creases create verticals on the bottom

NOW IT'S YOUR TURN

Flip through the Style Guide pages starting on page 35 and "go shopping." Pick out your most flattering tops (+) and see how they will combine with not only your flattering pants and skirts, but also with detracting (−) lower garments. Choose tops and jackets that can be worn as layers over (−) garments, thus turning them into a more positive (+) look.

Add (+)s to a (−) to Get (+)

When you are considering buying an item, check the Style Guide to see if any of your figure problems are circled under the illustration of that style.

If a garment is a (−) for part of your figure, look through the Style Guide to find a (+) garment you can wear with it. Combine them, like the examples below, to create an ensemble that is totally figure flattering.

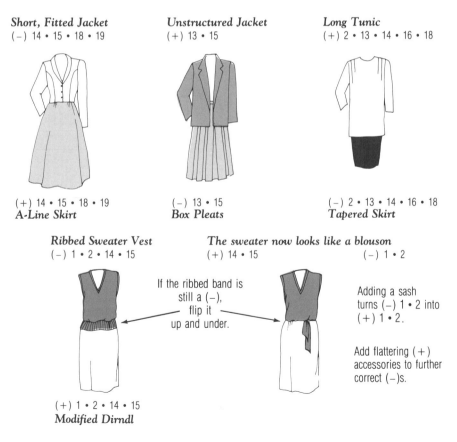

Short, Fitted Jacket
(−) 14 • 15 • 18 • 19

Unstructured Jacket
(+) 13 • 15

Long Tunic
(+) 2 • 13 • 14 • 16 • 18

(+) 14 • 15 • 18 • 19
A-Line Skirt

(−) 13 • 15
Box Pleats

(−) 2 • 13 • 14 • 16 • 18
Tapered Skirt

Ribbed Sweater Vest
(−) 1 • 2 • 14 • 15

The sweater now looks like a blouson
(+) 14 • 15

(−) 1 • 2

If the ribbed band is still a (−), flip it up and under.

Adding a sash turns (−) 1 • 2 into (+) 1 • 2.

Add flattering (+) accessories to further correct (−)s.

(+) 1 • 2 • 14 • 15
Modified Dirndl

★ **CONCEPT:** Salvage detracting (−) styles by combining them with flattering (+) styles.

SPECIAL STRATEGIES FOR MAXIMIZING YOUR POTENTIAL

Underneath It All

Illusions begin with your posture and what you wear under your clothes. Properly selected and fitted undergarments can make an amazing difference in how you look.

POSTURE. Good posture telegraphs self-confidence. Stand tall, throw those shoulders back, tuck that tummy in, take a deep breath, and smile. You will look better without spending a cent!

BRA TEST. Even small-busted women need to do this test in front of a mirror. Place the stick and string as illustrated.

The space between the base of your neck (find the two little bones) and your waist is all the space you have for a bosom. The fullest part of the bosom should be no lower than halfway in-between. Look in a mirror and see if your bosom is closer to your waist. If so, you need a new bra!

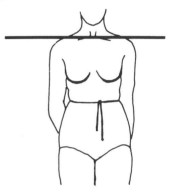

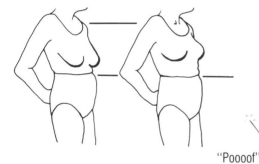

Adjust your bra straps to lift your low or full bosom to midchest. (Many women think they are short waisted when they are just low bosomed!)

A younger—and thinner looking you!

"Poooof"

When your bra fits correctly, clothes will fit better, too.

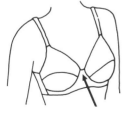

TRAMPOLINE TEST. To find out if your bra is properly fitted, do the "Trampoline Test:" Place your finger on your bra in the cleavage area and push.

If your finger can bounce in and out (as if it is jumping on a trampoline), you are *not* properly fitted. Next, feel along the edge of your bra in the front and down the seam under your arm. Are there any bulges? If so, you need a larger cup. The cup size—A, B, C, etc.—refers to the size of your bosom, the number—32, 36, 40—refers to the proper size of your rib cage. A properly fitted bra should touch your chest at the sternum (cleavage) and support your bosom at midchest without any bulges.

FABRICS: WEIGHTS AND VOLUME

The crispness or draping properties of a fabric also effect how your figure is camouflaged or revealed. In Chapter 3 on page 30, the same woman is shown in three very different silhouettes. Notice how a crisper fabric (1) creates volume while the knit garment (3) drapes and hugs her body shape. The medium suit-weight fabric (2) is concealing her body contours rather than revealing every curve. Be aware that shiny fabrics such as satin will both cling and reflect even the most minor figure curve.

Do avoid wearing thick, bulky fabrics where *you* are "bulky." Example: If you are "top-heavy," combine a lightweight blouse with a heavier-weight skirt or fuller slacks as shown in A.

Let your fabrics help you create visual balance.

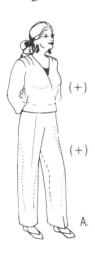

(+)

(+)

A.

A. A loose surplice-styled top (+) worn with loose, wide leg slacks (+) creates better visual balance for a heavy upper torso than a loose top worn with tight pants.

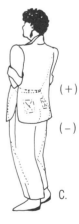

(+)

(−)

C.

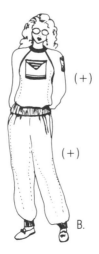

(+)

(+)

(+)

B.

B. This tall, too-thin body is enhanced by adding volume with thick knit fabric. The bulky fabric and horizontal design lines minimize her height and make her appear less "twiggy."

C. A crisp unstructured shirt (+) camouflages a heavy lower torso when worn over (−) hip-hugging jeans.

PRINT ME LARGER OR SMALLER

Plaids, prints, florals, lace, and knitted texture on sweaters can also assist you in creating illusions. Do the three-second Blink Test on these skirts to clarify the most dominant direction of prints and textures.

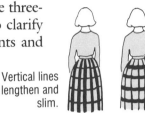

Vertical lines lengthen and slim.

Horizontal lines make you look wider.

Choose your plaids carefully according to which part of your torso you wish to widen or lengthen.

Prints may be mixed effectively if they:

- Are color coordinated
- Vary in size (mix small with medium; medium with large)

Wear the larger print where you want people to focus and the smaller print where you want to minimize attention.

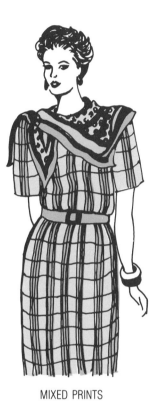

MIXED PRINTS

PRINT SIZE VS. YOUR SIZE

Who should wear large or small prints?

_____True_____False. Large women should not wear large prints.

I hope you answered false, because they can. Look at a print and notice if the shapes "bump" into each other or overlap. The *space between the shapes* will make a greater difference in how large you look than the actual size of the shapes. The following three illustrations show the same style made up in three types of floral prints. Notice how the eye follows the line of the flowers in A while it jumps from flower to flower in B, and in C you see the whole dress all at once. If you are large, choose A or C

★ **CONCEPT: An overall print can camouflage figure problems or detracting (−) style lines in clothing.**

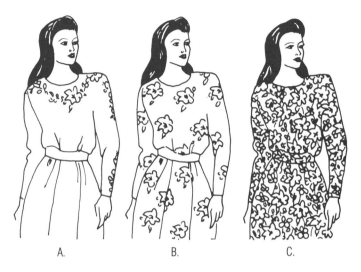

A.   B.   C.

Note: The flower shapes are the same size.

Tip: Wear prints near your figure assets, because prints are usually more eye-catching than a solid color.

PRINT SIZE VS. COLOR

Consider the size and color of prints in relation to *your* size and coloring.

Q. What size and color of prints come to mind when you visualize a 5 foot, 3 inch Hawaiian woman with black hair and bronzed skin?

A. Bold, BIG florals; intense, bright colors.

Q. What size and color of prints come to mind when you visualize a 5 foot, 6 inch British woman with pale blond hair and fair skin?

A. Tweeds and small florals; soft, subdued colors.

Try mentally dressing the Hawaiian woman in a blended, subdued English tweed. Now envision the taller fair British woman in a big, vivid Hawaiian print. Both would be a visual disaster. Why? Because the color intensities and the print sizes do not relate to their natural body colors.

GENERAL COLOR GUIDELINES. Regardless of your size, the stronger your body colors (skin and hair) are, the brighter your wardrobe colors should be and the bolder your prints may be. Softer body coloring is enhanced with softer wardrobe colors and more blended prints. More than your height or your weight, your body coloring is the key when selecting the print size and color intensity that will enhance you.

Color is critical in appearing healthy and glowing. If you hear how tired, rather than how terrific, you look, it is probably the lack of flattering colors and/or makeup. If you are wearing a garment that is fabulous for your figure and fits perfectly but you still are not getting compliments, it is probably due to the garment's color. Many of the professionals who teach *FYF* classes also offer color and makeup assistance. Request their names by using the "Would You Like More Information" form on page 101. Flattering colors and flattering styles are always a winning combination!

COLOR ME TALLER

Don't limit your use of color in an attempt to look taller. Color combinations A, B, C, and D may be used by women of *any* height.
★ **CONCEPT: To appear taller, combine colors that are similar in value (lightness or darkness).**

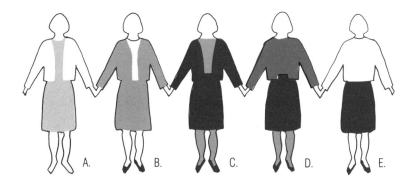

A. Inside garments all one color. **Concept:** Combine two light colors.
B. Outside garments all one color.
C. One color neck to toe maximizes height, but will not make you appear that much taller than options A, B, or D.
D. **Concept:** Combine medium with dark colors.
E. Light and dark color combinations do shorten the body.
Hosiery colors: Matching hose to hemline and shoe colors elongates legs, compare D and E.

SUIT ME SLIMMER

Do you ever try on a garment and wonder why you instantly look heavier? It could be the buttons! Study how the jackets below affect the thickness of a torso. While her waist and hips are drawn *exactly the same* width in each style, the changes in the hemlines and the positions of the buttons create the illusion of being thicker or slimmer. Notice how the angle of the points makes you look either down (B) or across (C) her hips.

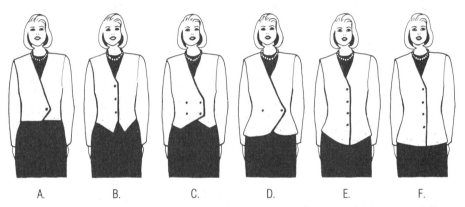

A.   B.   C.   D.   E.   F.

Beware: Even women with great figures can sabotage their potential when style lines add weight visually.

FIT ME LOOSE

Check for ease in the fit of a garment.

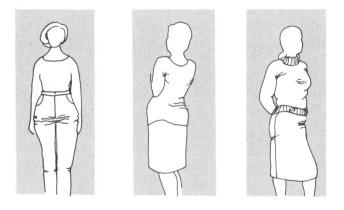

Wrinkles create horizontal lines!!

Tops and dresses: Raise arms; then lower; if the garment gets "stuck" on any part of you, try the next size. Avoid spreading lapels and pleats and straining button closures.

Skirts and pants: Check by sitting down and then standing up. Does it bind across your legs as you sit or get stuck on the tummy or hips when you stand? If so, try the next size.

SIZE ME UP

As manufacturers do not label all sizes exactly the same way, the number on the tag is not as important as the way you look in the garment. A larger size that fits with ease will actually make you look slimmer. *Cut the size tag out* of the garment if the number on it bothers you!

Try proportioned clothing to get your best fit and look.

Petites (under 5 feet, 4 inches) and **Juniors:**
   Cut for shorter figures and torsos
Misses: Cut for "average" figures
Tall: Cut for 5 feet, 10 inches and over
Women's Petites/Half Sizes: Cut for the fuller figure

ACCENT YOUR ASSETS

Most minor and many major figure problems can be camouflaged; however, there are some that are just too obvious to be camouflaged completely. The solution? Create a *visual diversion* that is so eye-catching that people automatically look at your assets rather than at your problems.

You may feel like many women who have participated in *FYF* classes: eager to share all your negatives, but hesitant to acknowledge anything attractive about yourself. This is when it truly helps to have others assist you in evaluating your figure.

For example, a lovely full-figured lady attended one of my classes. When we asked her to share her positive points, she looked down and, with a shake of her head, remained silent. (I later learned that her negative self-esteem was based on years of criticism by her family about her weight.)

I asked the other women to share what they saw as her potential assets. Within seconds we had a wonderful list. When I mentioned her legs, it was just too much for her to accept. With an explosive "Legs!" she jumped up and yanked up her skirt to reveal her thighs. Now, I have to admit that her thighs were not an area to accent, but I asked her to lower her skirt and look at her lower leg, which was beautifully shaped with tapered ankles—definitely attractive. "Just because part of your leg is not terrific doesn't mean that you have to reject the entire leg," I told her. We discussed how she could accent her great-looking lower legs. Soon we had a list that included wearing hosiery that was patterned, textured, or with seams that would cause people to look at her legs, not her hips. especially from the back. Shoes with interesting details or colors would also call attention to her legs, as would the hemlines of skirts such as these:

HEMLINES AND BORDERS THAT ACCENT LEGS

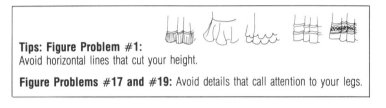

Tips: Figure Problem #1:
Avoid horizontal lines that cut your height.

Figure Problems #17 and #19: Avoid details that call attention to your legs.

COUNT YOUR BLESSINGS

The moment of truth has arrived! Yes, you are going to be asked to say something nice about yourself. Don't let modesty be an obstacle. It's time to identify your assets and then—FLAUNT THEM!
List three of your best features here. (One may be above your neck).

———————————————————————————

———————————————————————————

———————————————————————————

Are you drawing a blank? Think about any compliments you have received—even old ones. If you get stuck, ask your friends, family, or a professional what parts of your body have the highest potential to become an asset—then don't discount or deny their answers. Look in the mirror and see what they see. Get used to compliments—you will soon be hearing them more often. Think positively about your assets. Learn to compliment yourself!

Turn to your (+) Figure Assets (+) chart on page 99 and follow the directions in identifying your best features. Where are your assets? How can you direct attention to them? The following sections will give you some clues.

FOCAL POINTS

A focal point is created when you divert a viewer's attention to a specific spot.

The best example I can think of to illustrate this is the moment when I met my husband—by a swimming pool. Now, swimwear reveals more than it conceals and calls for major diversion tactics. Thank goodness I was wearing an enormous floppy straw hat. He remembered me as the woman in the hat rather than "Jell-O thighs!"

Observe how each change creates a different Focal Point on this outfit.

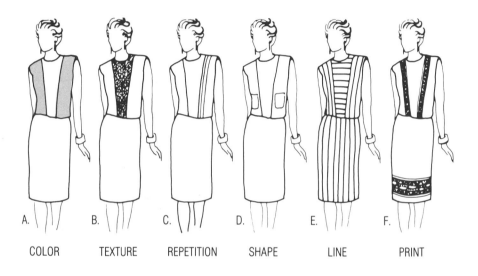

A.   B.   C.   D.   E.   F.

COLOR   TEXTURE   REPETITION   SHAPE   LINE   PRINT

A small change in a style can create a focal point on your . . .

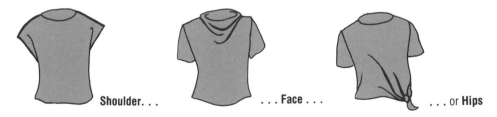

Shoulder. . .   . . . **Face** . . .   . . . or **Hips**

Practice the Blink Test on the four ensembles below. Cover the illustrations you are not testing, leaving only one revealed. Close your eyes; then open them. Instantly: where do you look first? *Circle* the Focal Point and determine why your "instant impression" focused there. The answers are below.

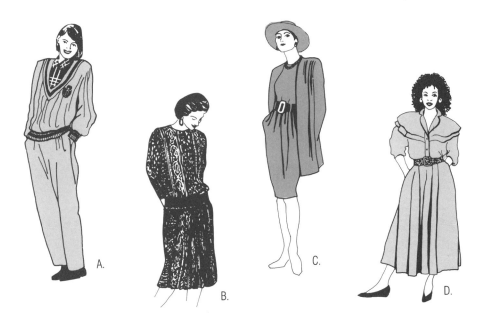

Tip: If your answers are incorrect, have a friend hold your workbook 2 to 3 feet away and do the Blink Test again. The Focal Point of the style is the one seen from a distance.

FOCAL POINT	PART OF BODY	WHY
A. Shirt/V-neck	Face/neck	Pattern on solid color
B. Drop-waist band	Hips	Solid color on pattern
C. Big belt buckle	Waist	Shiny metal is eye-catching
D. "Cape"	Shoulders	Distinctive style lines

Turn to the "(+) Style Lines That Flatter My Figure (+)" section of your Figure Chart (page 99). Compare the lines on your chart to the style lines on the four outfits above. Are the lines of these garments flattering for you?

A. Diverging/vertical lines near the face; horizontal line on the hips.
B. Horizontal line on the hips.
C. Horizontal line at the waist; vertical jacket lines.
D. Horizontal lines at the bust and waist.

DIVERSION

When a detracting style line cannot be corrected or camouflaged, use Focal Points to minimize detracting (−) parts of the style by diverting attention toward the more flattering (+) parts of it and you. For example, if the cape in D above is a minus (−) on you, you could change the belt to a contrasting color and divert attention from the upper torso and toward the waist.

ACCESSORIES

A fun and easy way to create Focal Points is with accessories. Let's start with the necessary accessories, such as your leather items.

SHOE SAVVY

A basic shoe wardrobe includes casual to dressy shoes plus boots and sports shoes, as needed for your lifestyle. The shoe chart on page 78 shows silhouettes of such a variety. Notice how as the heels get lower and thicker, the shoe looks heavier and more casual, while the higher and thinner the heel, the lighter and dressier it looks.

Shoe Colors

The best shoe colors for you to invest in are your own natural body colors: your hair and skin tone. No matter what clothing colors you put on, you are always wearing your body colors. Repeat them on your feet! Wearing your hair color as a shoe color creates color balance from head to toe.

By acquiring a few basic shoes in your natural body colors, you will always have a shoe to complement both you and your wardrobe. Add other styles and colors from the different sections of the shoe chart as your budget allows.

Shoe and Hosiery Tips

- Shoe and hose colors that match the main color of your hemline will make your legs look longer.
- The color of your shoes may differ from the color of your handbag so long as both compliment your total ensemble . . . and you.
- Hose color should not be darker than shoe color.

- Dark sheer hosiery "shadows" and slims legs; pale hosiery enlarges legs.
- Wooden heels are never dressy.
- Ankle straps, T-straps, and high vamps will make your leg look shorter.
- Your hemline should cover the top of your boot. Leaving a gap between them creates a negative focal point and visually shortens your leg.

Put Your Best Foot Forward

The complex lifestyles of many women require a diverse clothing and shoe wardrobe. Cover half of the model's image in the illustration below. Which shoe styles will enhance each of her images? (Hint: There may be more than one answer.)

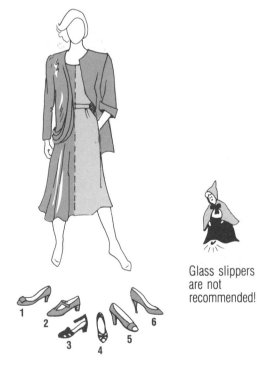

Glass slippers are not recommended!

Answers to the Shoe Selection quiz

Dressy style: 1, 4, or 6
Business/day dress: 1, 5, or 6

Closed-toe pumps of solid colored leather like 1 and 6 are excellent investments that complement a variety of outfits.

SHOE CHART

STYLE (Weight)	FLAT	MEDIUM HEEL	HIGH HEEL	BOOT (Heavyweight)
CASUAL Light				
Medium				
Heavy		Espadrille	Wedge	
		Clog		
DAY DRESS BUSINESS Light				**(Medium weight)**
Medium		Louis Heel	Slingback	
Heavy		T-Strap	Pump	
		Spectator		
		Wooden Heel		**Concepts:** Wear lower, thicker heels and soles with casual clothes and thicker fabrics (wool, denim, and cotton knits).
DRESSY Light		Slide	Anklestrap	Wear higher, thinner heels and soles with dressy garments made of lightweight fabrics (silk, chiffon, and cotton batiste).
			Spike Heel	

Heel Height vs. Skirt Length

The length of your skirt, the length of your leg, and the height of your heel are all seen as a unit. Try on three different heel heights (flat, midheel, and high heel) with the longest skirt or dress you own; then try them with your shortest skirt. You will see that the different heel heights affect your entire look. Make notes of the combinations that flatter your leg shape, length, and your total height.

Tip for Figure Problem #1 and Short Women: Avoid wearing extra long skirts with flats—and looking like you are standing in a hole!

WHAT'S IN THE BAG, LADY?

It seems I always get stuck in lines behind a woman who has lost her wallet in the depths of a giant bag. I think handbags are like closets: the larger they are, the more you stuff into them. When I use handbags from the audience during workshops demonstrations, I am overwhelmed by the amount and weight of items women carry around all day.

All too often a mismatched handbag ruins what could be a fabulous look. I challenge you to change handbags to complement your total image, each time you get dressed. Take the hassle out of changing handbags by following these steps:

1. Dump everything in the last handbag you used into a basket or box.
2. Select a handbag that is complementary to your current outfit (see the handbag chart).
3. Put in it *only* the items you will need between the time you leave home and the time you return.
4. When you return home, empty your handbag into the basket before putting it away.
5. Repeat these steps every time you get dressed.

This makes it easy to select the best bag for each outfit. Just think, you will never again have to search through your bags to find lost lipstick or keys—they are in the basket!

HANDBAG CHART

Image	Size	Materials	Typical Features
Sporty, casual	Medium to large	Hard leathers Canvas, Vinyl Straw, Mesh, Plastic	Combination of materials Plastic handle Shoulder straps
Business	Briefcase	Leather Padded vinyl	Hand grip or shoulder strap Box shape
Day	Wide variety	Soft leather and Suede Reptile/skins	Metal clasp Leather, metal or bone handle
Dressy	Medium to small	Very soft leather Nice fabrics	Leather or Metal handle
Evening	Small to tiny	Elegant fabrics Tapestry Formed metals	Beaded Metallic Shiny

Turn back to the illustrations on page 30. Would you have an appropriate handbag for each of the outfits?

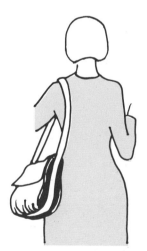

Can't Find Your Keys? Put personal items in a small clutch. Put clutch into tote or briefcase.

Tip: Your handbag should contain only the items necessary while you are out.

Beware! Bulky bags broaden!

Handbag Hints

- If you are carrying the same handbag with every outfit, it will often detract ($-$) from rather than complement ($+$) your ensemble.
- Handbags that are multicolored, textured, shiny, or patterned may create Focal Points.
- Color coordinate your bag to your garments, accessories, or your own skin and hair colors.
- When you need a large carryall, put your personal items in a small clutch; put the clutch into your tote or briefcase.
- Just because a handbag has a high price tag does not mean that it is dressy. Outrageously expensive designer bags made with heavy, thick leather straps combined with vinyl are *very* casual. Be sure that the pattern on the bag—even if it is the designer's name—complements rather than competes with your garments or prints.
- Fashion names change with time: Your grandmother carried a pocketbook, your mother carried a purse, you carry a handbag!
- Shorten shoulder bag straps: Avoid wearing bulky bags where you are bulky!

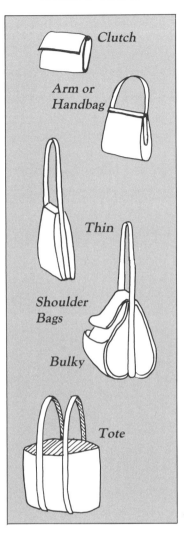

Clutch

Arm or Handbag

Thin

Shoulder Bags

Bulky

Tote

BELTS FOR EVERY BODY

To belt, not to belt, or how to belt are often the questions. If you have a definite waist, *do* wear belts, even if your weight is not ideal (see the test for Wide Waist, page 25). Follow these tips for Figure Problems #2, 11, 13, 14, and 15:

Minimize attention on your waist by:

- Wearing small narrow belts, fastened loosely
- Selecting belt colors that blend with the garment color
- Avoiding reflective metals, materials, and metal buckles

Caution to all: Belting your waist to look smaller may make your hips or bustline look proportionately larger!

Circle all of your Major figure problem numbers under the following illustrations to discover your best belt styles and placement.

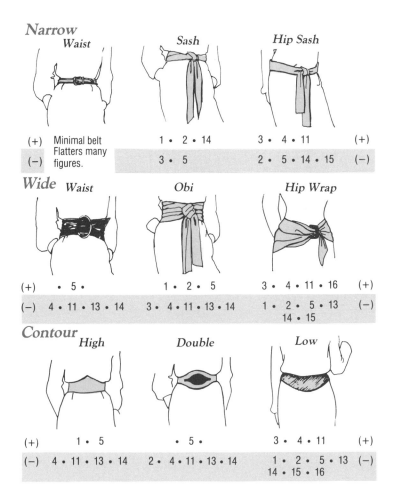

Narrow

	Waist	Sash	Hip Sash	
(+)	Minimal belt Flatters many	1 • 2 • 14	3 • 4 • 11	(+)
(−)	figures.	3 • 5	2 • 5 • 14 • 15	(−)

Wide

	Waist	Obi	Hip Wrap	
(+)	• 5 •	1 • 2 • 5	3 • 4 • 11 • 16	(+)
(−)	4 • 11 • 13 • 14	3 • 4 • 11 • 13 • 14	1 • 2 • 5 • 13 14 • 15	(−)

Contour

	High	Double	Low	
(+)	1 • 5	• 5 •	3 • 4 • 11	(+)
(−)	4 • 11 • 13 • 14	2 • 4 • 11 • 13 • 14	1 • 2 • 5 • 13 14 • 15 • 16	(−)

NECK ACCESSORIES

Necklines, accessories, and face shapes are seen as a unit. Notice how the accessories below dominate the necklines. They have the power to change a detracting (−) neckline to a flattering (+) one. Use your accessories to salvage any neckline that is circled as a minus (−) for you.

Circle your figure problem numbers under these styles to discover how to use neck accessories to accent you!

High: Flattering for long necks.

Necklaces	*Ties*	*Scarves*

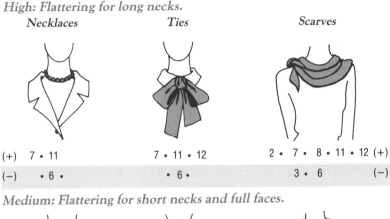

(+) 7 • 11	7 • 11 • 12	2 • 7 • 8 • 11 • 12 (+)
(−) • 6 •	• 6 •	3 • 6 (−)

Medium: Flattering for short necks and full faces.

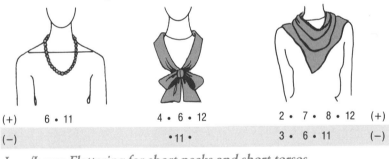

(+) 6 • 11	4 • 6 • 12	2 • 7 • 8 • 12 (+)
(−)	•11•	3 • 6 • 11 (−)

Low/Long: Flattering for short necks and short torsos.

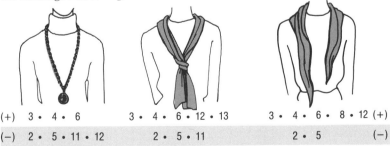

(+) 3 • 4 • 6	3 • 4 • 6 • 12 • 13	3 • 4 • 6 • 8 • 12 (+)
(−) 2 • 5 • 11 • 12	2 • 5 • 11	2 • 5 (−)

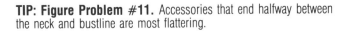

TIP: Figure Problem #11. Accessories that end halfway between the neck and bustline are most flattering.

Flattering Your Figure—Today **83**

PROPORTION AND PERSONAL STYLE

In selecting accessories, proportion is important: as shoulder pads got larger, so did earrings, even for small women.

CONCEPT: The size of your accessories should increase in proportion to the size of your body and/or garments.

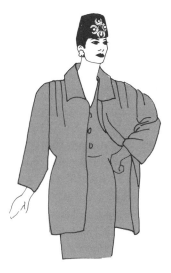

Tip: A hat should "fit your figure" as well as your head!

Rather than looking fashionable, the tiny hat combined with the voluminous outfit looks ridiculous. Check any hat purchase by doing the Blink Test (pages 89–90) in front of a full-length mirror.

Use the concepts of vertical and horizontal lines with your earrings and scarves. And remember: Repetition of a shape emphasizes it. Compare the effect of longer earrings and necklace to the repetition of round jewelry on a round face on page 34.

Earrings are great for creating visual diversions. It is hard to focus on any figure problems when a woman wears an unusual, dangling, or large earring!

Accessories can turn the "blahs" into personality, polish, or . . . pizzazz! Your choices of jewelry, scarves, or a hat are true expressions of your own individual personality. How many different personal statements can be created from the basic dress and the accessories on the next page? Which of the accessory combinations would you choose to wear?

PERSONAL STYLE

Select five accessories to create each of these personal styles:
  • Classic • Romantic • Dramatic • Arty • Sporty.

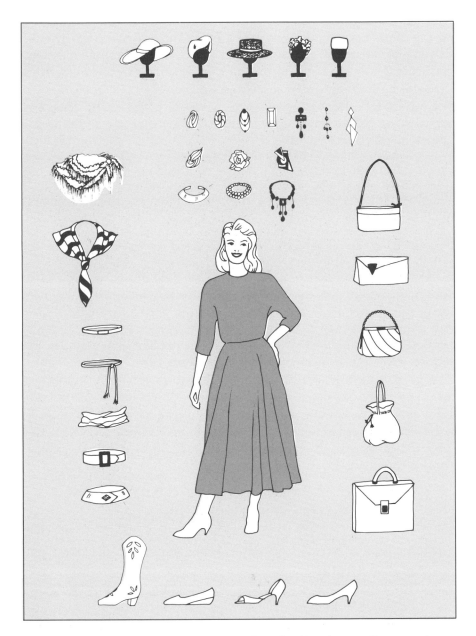

(Now you know why this woman is smiling—and travels with only one suitcase on a two-week trip!)

UP TO YOUR NECK IN ACCESSORIES

Take stock of your neck accessories. What additions would be your best investments? Place five of your favorite skirts or slacks on your bed. Now lay a scarf, necklace, or pin that repeats the color of the garment on top of each one. Make a shopping list of the colors you are missing. Acquire a variety of accessories that match the color of your *lower* garments. Have fun wearing the color-matched garments and accessories with a variety of different colored tops.

CONCEPT: Repeating next to your face the color that you are wearing below your waist is an easy way to create a wonderful, color-coordinated ensemble.

Color Tip: Repeat an accent color with several accessories such as red belt, shoes, and earrings . . . or purple blouse, belt, and handbag.

How many accessories should you wear? As many as your heart desires! Although accessory trends swing from minimal to many, how many you choose to wear should reflect your own personality. I once had an art history professor who averaged fourteen pieces of jewelry per day. Unusual? Yes. Distinctive? Yes! She remains a very unique and unforgettable visual memory even twenty years later.

A word of caution: While you may choose to wear any number of accessories for your social and personal life, conservative is the word in many businesses. A noisy set of bracelets, fingers covered with rings, or large dangling earrings can be distracting in business meetings. Observe the garments and accessories your female superiors are wearing as a guide to what is acceptable in your office.

FLATTER YOUR FIGURE SUMMARY

- Camouflage and correct figure problems with styles that are a plus (+) for your figure.
- Camouflage detracting (–) styles by combining them with flattering (+) styles that are more noticeable.
- Divert attention from figure or clothing problems that you cannot camouflage. Direct it instead toward your assets by using colors, prints, and accessories.

CHAPTER
5

Mirror, Mirror, on the Wall

"They aren't making mirrors the way they used to."
—Tallulah Bankhead

Confidence. That is the feeling you get when you know that you really look great. Compliments from others are confirmation of that feeling. Unfortunately, years of figure and fashion frustrations have robbed many women of both compliments and confidence. It is very disheartening to spend extra effort—and money—putting together what you think is a great outfit, only to wear it and never receive even a comment.

Do you wonder, like so many of the women who attend *Flatter Your Figure* classes, "How can I *really* know that my outfit compliments me?" Here is the answer.

HOW TO READ AN IMAGE

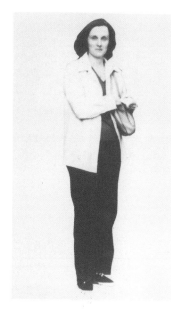

What is an image? An image is the total impression created by a person. It encompasses your body, your clothing, your posture, and even your attitude.

Study the woman in this photograph and answer the questions below.

1. She is about _____ years old.
2. She completed _____ years of formal education.
3. She is employed as a _____ _____ or _____.
4. Her annual salary is $_____.
5. Will she get a raise or promotion this year? Yes   No
6. Her self-esteem is _____.

If you guessed that this is a picture of Jan Larkey when she was 4-F—forty, fat, faded, and frumpy—you are right. This is the photograph, mentioned in Chapter 1, that shocked me into changing my image. Compare my image to the actual facts and my picture on the back cover. The answers to the Jan Larkey quiz are:

1. Forty
2. Master's degree from Stanford University
3. Job hunting: Art Teacher
4. Previous salary: $15,000 (1980)
5. Standard raise—if teaching!
6. Low self-esteem: 4-F!

Every time anyone sees you, you are being "interviewed." Whether it is for a job, a friendship, or a life partner, your appearance sends a loud and clear message, even when you are silent. It shows the people in your life how you value yourself . . . and them.

My outside image was sending a dismal message that did not invite anyone to meet the woman inside.

What message is your image sending?

SENDING MIXED MESSAGES

On city streets, the sight of a business suit combined with jogging shoes is so jarring that your eyes instantly focus on the feet—and stay there. This is an obvious "mixed image message" that hits a discordant visual note and is easy to spot.

What is hard to spot is a more subtle mixed message: the earring that is too delicate for the sports outfit, the shiny belt buckle that becomes an unintentional focal point, or the thick heel that looks too heavy for the flowing skirt.

We know that seeing yourself as others see you is not always easy. Yet I discovered a fascinating way to see yourself clearly with the blink of your eyes. Yes, it's the same Blink Test that you have been practicing on style lines, pattern directions, and focal points.

When I started my make-over, I wanted a quick and objective way to evaluate if what I was wearing really complimented me. I experimented until I discovered that standing back away from a mirror allowed me to get a better perspective on my whole body. Then, if I blinked slowly and blocked out my image, what I saw when I opened my eyes was an "instant snapshot" of myself.

To find out what message your own image is sending and to see yourself as others (and cameras) see you, test your image impact every time you get dressed by doing . . .

THE BLINK TEST

1. Stand *at least 5 feet* from a full-length mirror. Close your eyes. Count to three.
2. Open your eyes. *Instantly:* What do you see first? Your assets? Your figure problems? Do *you and all the parts of your wardrobe* look good together?

What you see first is what others will also notice first. If anything strikes a jarring note when you open your eyes, change it, especially if it calls attention to a problem area. Repeat the Blink Test, making changes until you see your positive points immediately and a harmonious total image.

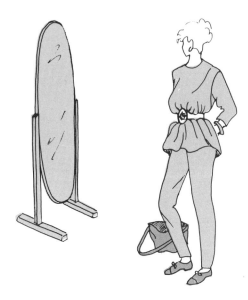

Jarring Notes:
  Tight belt, Low bra
Make changes until you . . .

PASS YOUR BLINK TEST. YOU'LL LOVE THE RESULTS!

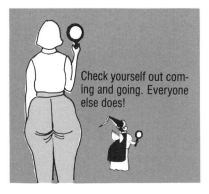

Check yourself out coming and going. Everyone else does!

Tsk. . .Tsk. . .Tsk. . .
Head for the skirt racks!

Note: Too many women look only from the neck down when trying on clothes. If your face disappears when you do the Blink Test, it is time to learn how to flatter yourself from the neck up . . . hmmmm . . . that sounds like a good topic for another book. . . . If you have other image-related problems that concern you, please let me know by sending in the form on page 101. As an author, I want to write about what you want to know . . . this is your chance to tell me!

GOOD, BETTER, BEST

To gain further practice in reading an image, do the Blink Test on the following illustrations.

How many things can you find wrong with the two images below? Circle each detracting (−) problem. What would you change or add to make her ensembles have head-to-toe harmony?

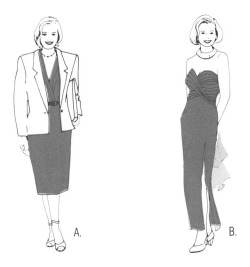

A. Her message is mixed: half of her image looks ready for work, the other half seems to be looking for a party. Secure the blouse opening higher and have the suit jacket altered—it swallows her. The delicate jewelry and flirtatious shoes both need to be changed.

B. This shoe style and heel would look more appropriate with the suit than this elegant, sheer evening gown. Try switching the jewelry and shoes between A and B. Both ensembles will then send a clear message from hairstyle to shoe: one means business, the other says social.

LEARN FROM OTHER PEOPLE'S SUCCESSES

Do the Blink Test when you see a smashing-looking outfit on a woman (or on a mannequin). Study how the wardrobe pieces were combined and what was used to create the Focal Points. This is a great way to train your eye to analyze the impact of clothing on figures. (If people ask if you have something in your eye, just smile and tell them you're, "FOoooOF-ing!")

SUCCESS AT LAST

The very first time I tried the Blink Test I saw many things that needed to be corrected. Just changing my handbag made a big improvement. Each time I did the Blink Test, my understanding of what I needed to do to improve my image increased . . . so did my self-confidence. What a great feeling! I still remember the outfit I was wearing the first time I blinked and finally did not have to change one thing. Soon, I was passing my Blink Test more and more often. I was finally in control of my appearance.

Learning how to correct a lifetime of shopping and dressing mistakes and pass the Blink Test consistently wasn't instantaneous. (Be patient. Acquiring a closet full of figure-flattering clothes does take time!) But, at last, I had a foolproof way to evaluate my dressing decisions. Getting dressed became an adventure and a challenge rather than a frustrating and depressing daily chore. I soon discovered that "playing dress-up" can be fun, even at age forty, when the results turn negative feelings into smiles. No more 4-F feelings for me!

EXCUSES, EXCUSES, EXCUSES

It is one thing to dislike your image and not know how to change it. It is another thing to know how to look great and choose not to. Some favorite excuses for looking 4-F are

I DON'T HAVE TIME. Passing your Blink Test, like any skill, will take a few extra minutes in the beginning. Every time you change something, you are learning what does, or does not, enhance you (thus saving time forever after). Spending ten extra minutes to look good for ten hours is time well spent! Keep experimenting. You will soon be able to create a positive image quickly.

SPECIAL EVENTS. You may be thinking, I'll do the Blink Test when I get dressed up to go somewhere special. Aren't you special? Every day? Even if you live the most casual of lifestyles, with jeans and sweatshirts as your staple wardrobe, apply the *FYF* concepts for selecting and wearing them. You can look terrific—or terrible—in casual clothes. Keep in mind that "casual" and "sloppy" are not synonyms!

MONEY AND MOTHERHOOD. Some women use excuses for not looking terrific such as: "There isn't enough money, I'll do without" or "The children need so much; I can wait." Money and the needs of others are not the issues. Your self-esteem is. Flattering clothing choices are available at all price levels. You don't need an extensive or expensive wardrobe to eliminate a negative image. What you and your family truly need is a mother, wife, and woman who radiates positive feelings about herself.

LOOKING GOOD VS. VANITY. We are admonished to love others as we love ourselves. How loved would your friends feel if you said to them some of the disparaging comments you make to yourself when you look in a mirror? The *FYF* system does not advocate narcissism or vanity, but a healthy attitude toward fulfilling your potential and looking the best you can. Seeing your reflection and feeling positive about your image contributes to a wholesome feeling.

A SPECIAL NOTE FOR TEENS

As a teenager, one of the most important criteria for what you choose to wear is what your friends are wearing. Conferring on clothes and making sure that your outfit is acceptable at your school and social events may be much more important than dressing to flatter your figure. You can do both. If you follow the trends of your friends in buying your wardrobe pieces, follow the tips in this book on how you can put them together to make your figure look good too.

The teens below are all dressed in the same basic pieces, yet each one has done something different with her collar, shirttails, and legs to flatter her figure challenges:

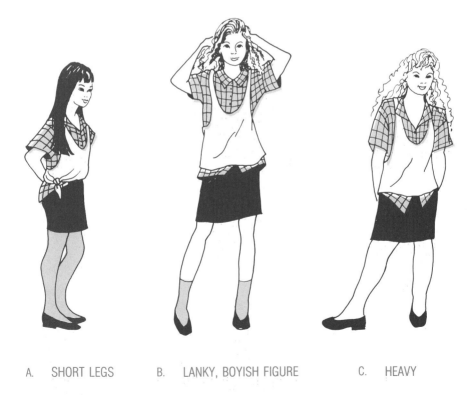

A. SHORT LEGS   B. LANKY, BOYISH FIGURE   C. HEAVY

A SPECIAL NOTE FOR MOTHERS OF TEENAGERS

It has been my personal experience that letting my children (currently aged thirty-one, twenty-eight, and seventeen) make their own decisions during their teen years about what to buy and wear has saved me a tremendous amount of time, money, and frustration. While you may shudder at what your teenagers are wearing, they are friend-focused and your objections will probably result in minimal changes and maximum resentment. Be patient. By age nineteen or twenty they will rediscover their individuality, and they may even ask for your opinion about their wardrobe.

Being asked to go to the mall with my teenage daughter is a treat. The only catch is that to avoid embarrassment, she wants to pick out what *I* wear. So, if you see me shopping in baggy pants pegged at the ankles, an oversize T-shirt, super-sprayed-up hair, and no lipstick—the cute blond with me is my daughter!

SEVEN SECONDS TO IMAGE IMPACT

Research shows that you have only seven seconds to make a first impression. Professionally, your image may determine if *you* get the job—and it may even affect your salary level. If you are getting great performance reviews but are passed up for promotions, your image may be the cause.

Creating a positive first impression can pay off personally too. Consider again the fairy tale of Cinderella. It was her charm and personality (what is on the inside) that captivated the prince—but only after her gorgeous (and appropriate) ballgown got her through the palace doors. Although clothes alone cannot ensure success in the ballroom or the boardroom, they do open or close doors of opportunity. Like it or not, we are initially judged by our "cover."

For some of you, applying the information in this book may be the start of a head-to-toe make-over; for others, *FYF* may make the more subtle differences between looking good, better, and best. For each of you it can mean an increase in self-confidence. It doesn't matter whether you are casually dressed for a trip to the grocery store or elegantly attired for the opera, the inner glow that starts with a smile as you pass your Blink Test is there for all to sense.

Looking your best means never having to make excuses about your appearance . . . especially to yourself.

IT'S UP TO YOU

This book was written for every woman who has a figure problem or who feels negative about her appearance. It was written for women like Abby.

Abby called one day several years after she had first come to me for assistance with her appearance. Through the years she participated in a variety of classes and workshops I offer on color, makeup, fashion, and figure problems. She shared with me a very personal experience.

Abby had become a member of Al-Anon, an organization for the families of alcoholics. Her first time to share her story with the support group had occurred the previous evening. After telling of the years of heartache, she shared what had happened that was positive in her life. She said, "For the first time in my life I feel put together. Jan Larkey put the outside of me together, and Al-Anon has put the inside together.

"Oh, Abby," I said, "What a wonderful compliment. But you are attributing your success to the wrong person. It was *you* who put yourself together. All I did was give you the guidelines to use. It was you who applied them and made the difference, not I."

Flatter Your Figure gives you the guidelines.

I hope you will choose to use them.

WHERE DO I START?

Start using the *FYF* system with some of the clothes you already own. Tonight, when you are getting undressed, try on two garments from your closet: one of your favorites and a "guilt garment" that you don't wear. Evaluate each style on your figure by doing the Blink Test (5 feet from your mirror.) Use the *Flatter Your Figure* Style Guide and your Figure Chart to help you understand why one is flattering, while the other is a mistake.

Next, have some fun. Experiment with layers and accessories. See if you can salvage the mistake—and make your favorite garment look even better.

Before today is over, you will have learned more about how the *Flatter Your Figure* concepts actually work on your own figure. You will be on your way to making better buying decisions; avoiding mistakes; saving time, money, and effort . . . and looking better.

MY THREE WISHES

If I could have three wishes granted, this is what they would be:

- My first wish is that every woman who feels frustrated about fashions or her figure would read this book. (Thank *you* for granting this wish. Please share it with your friends who express dressing room—or figure—despair.)
- My second wish is that each woman who reads *Flatter Your Figure* would be like Abby and really use it. I want you to get dressed and love the results—every day!
- My third wish is that you won't wait until tonight to try a figure-flattering idea. Do the Blink Test on what you are wearing. Make at least one change in the next few minutes that will improve your appearance for the rest of today.

. . . And don't forget—when you do the Blink Test—smile at the woman who decides how you look . . . YOU.

Because . . .

No woman is completely dressed until she wears a smile.
—Anonymous

Your Personal Figure Chart

HOW TO USE YOUR FIGURE CHART

To quickly evaluate if a garment will flatter your figure, do the Blink Test (pages 89–90) on it and answer these questions:

1. What *style line do you see first*? Compare *the direction of that line* to the lines that you drew on the figures. Does the direction of it follow any of your most flattering lines? See examples pages 31–33 and 64.

2. Where is the Focal Point (pages 74–75)? Does it focus attention on a spot you marked on your chart as a (+) Figure Asset (+)—or a (−) Figure Problem (−)?

When shopping, ordering, and sewing, keep in mind that perfect garments, like perfect bodies, rarely exist. Acquire garments that have the potential to become figure flattering when you apply the guidelines in this book.

Enjoy creating your own figure and wardrobe magic with clothing combinations that . . .

- Follow your most flattering (+) Style Lines (+)
- Minimize attention to your (−) Figure Problems (−)
- Focus attention on your (+) Figure Assets (+)

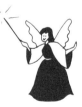

Exclusively Yours

Flatter Your Figure is now personalized for *YOUR FIGURE*. Take it shopping. Keep it in your closet or sewing area as a handy reference.

HOW TO COMPLETE YOUR FIGURE CHART

These directions are for completing the "Style Lines That Flatter My Figure" section on page 99.

Referring to the cover flap, circle your figure problem numbers below. Study the EXAMPLE below before drawing any vertical or horizontal lines on the figures in the style lines section of your chart.

If you have any of the problems listed below, draw VERTICAL lines on the figures (on the facing page) where each of your figure problems is located. Acquire clothing that emphasizes vertical lines on this area of the body.

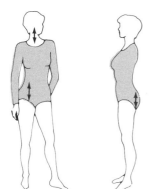

1	SHORT LEGS
2	WIDE HIPS
3	DOMINANT SHOULDERS
4	SHORT WAISTED
6	SHORT NECK • DOUBLE CHIN
10	HEAVY ARMS
11	FULL OR LOW BUST
13	WIDE WAIST
14	PROTRUDING ABDOMEN • SPARE TIRE
15	PROTRUDING DERRIERE • SWAYBACKED
18	LARGE THIGHS • SADDLEBAGS
19	LARGE CALVES • THICK ANKLES

Figure Problems:
↑ for #6, 14, and 15,
↓ and ←→ for #8

If you have any of the problems listed below, draw HORIZONTAL lines on the figures (on the facing page) where each of your figure problems is located. Acquire clothing that emphasizes horizontal lines on this area of the body.

5	LONG WAISTED
7	LONG NECK
8	ROUND/SLOPING SHOULDERS
9	THIN ARMS
12	SMALL BUST
16	FLAT DERRIERE
17	THIN LEGS

YOUR PERSONAL FIGURE CHART

(−) Figure Problems (−)

(Refer to the Cover Flap)

My figure problems are here:

Place a (−) on the figure below on the spot(s) where each of your Figure problems is located. Be sure that the problem is visually obvious to others.

(+) Figure Assets (+)

(Refer to page 73)

My assets are here:

Place a (+) on the figure below on the *three* most attractive parts of your figure (one may be above the neck.)

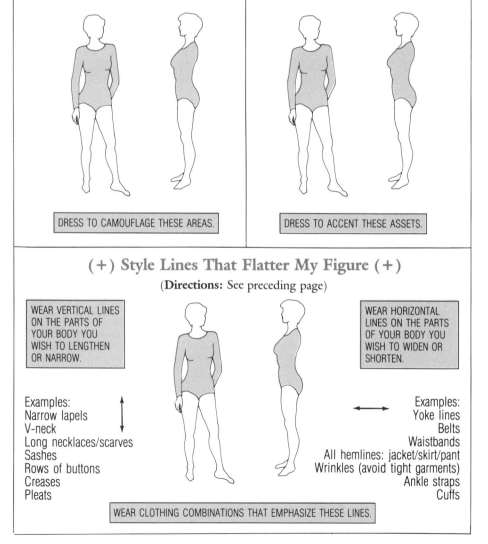

DRESS TO CAMOUFLAGE THESE AREAS.

DRESS TO ACCENT THESE ASSETS.

(+) Style Lines That Flatter My Figure (+)

(**Directions:** See preceding page)

WEAR VERTICAL LINES ON THE PARTS OF YOUR BODY YOU WISH TO LENGTHEN OR NARROW.

WEAR HORIZONTAL LINES ON THE PARTS OF YOUR BODY YOU WISH TO WIDEN OR SHORTEN.

Examples:
Narrow lapels
V-neck
Long necklaces/scarves
Sashes
Rows of buttons
Creases
Pleats

Examples:
Yoke lines
Belts
Waistbands
All hemlines: jacket/skirt/pant
Wrinkles (avoid tight garments)
Ankle straps
Cuffs

WEAR CLOTHING COMBINATIONS THAT EMPHASIZE THESE LINES.

Notes

WOULD YOU LIKE MORE INFORMATION?

To receive a *free* Shopping Tip Sheet complete this page (both sides), send it with a SASE (self-addressed, stamped, business-sized envelope) to:

Jan Larkey
FYF Survey
P.O. Box 8258
Pittsburgh, PA 15218

Name_____ Date_____

Street_____ Phone_____

City_____

State/Province _____ Country_____Zip_____

Please send me the name of the nearest professional who can:
_____ assist me personally.
_____ present a Flatter Your Figure™ program.

I NEED MORE HELP WITH:
_____ Makeup/Application   _____ Wardrobe Budgeting & Planning
_____ Hair Color/Style   _____ Wardrobe Coordination/Colors
_____ Selecting Eyeglasses   _____ Travel and Packing Tips
_____ Accessorizing   _____ Other _____

―――――――――――― Available Now ――――――――――――

"DRESSING TIPS that FLATTER YOUR FIGURE"
45 minute audio tape by Jan Larkey

Follow Jan's fun, informative step-by-step guide to creating new figure-flattering outfits from your own closet! Expands the ideas in *Flatter Your Figure®*. Discover how to organize your closet, salvage mistakes, plan your next purchases, and make dressing decisions quickly.
_____ Yes, please send me the "Dressing Tips" audio cassette tape.
Enclose $11.95 check or postal money order in US$, payable to JLIM.

INSTRUCTOR'S KIT available. Learn how to conduct *Flatter Your Figure®* consultations, classes, and programs.
_____ Please send me information about the FYF Instructor's Kit.
Or Call (412) 731-8558

MAKEUP AND HAIR PROBLEMS: A CONSUMER SURVEY

MAKEUP (Check the most appropriate answers)
I follow a skin care regime: ____ Daily ____ Frequently ____ Rarely
I use glamour cosmetics: ____ Daily ____ Frequently ____ Rarely
I have trouble ____ choosing makeup; ____ applying makeup.

What frustrates me the most about makeup is:

HAIR
My hair color is ____ natural ____ highlighted ____ colored.
When I ask for a "trim" I want my hair cut:
____ about ¼" ____ about ½" ____ about 1"
When I ask for a "cut" I want my hair cut:
____ less than 1" ____ about 1" ____ more than 1" ____ restyled
What frustrates me the most about my hair is:

FLATTER YOUR FIGURE® SURVEY

Please *circle* your Major figure problem numbers below.
  Underline your Minor figure problem numbers.

1 2 3 4 5 6 7 8 9 10 11 12 13 14 15 16 17 18 19

1. I would have liked more information about:

2. One of the most helpful things I learned from *Flatter Your Figure*® is:

Optional: ____ Yes, you may quote me. Signature _____

Thank you for your valuable information.